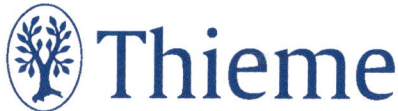

Imaging Handbook on Anatomy of Cochlea

Neeraj Suri, MS (ENT)
Associate Professor
ENT Department
GMERS Medical College
Gandhinagar, Gujarat

Thieme
Delhi • Stuttgart • New York • Rio de Janeiro

Publishing Director: Ritu Sharma
Developement Editor:
Dr. Astha Sawhney
Director Editorial Services:
Rachna Sinha
Project Manager: Deepanshu Manral
National Sales Manager:
Bishwajit Kumar Mishra
Managing Director & CEO: Ajit Kohli

Thieme Medical and Scientific
Publishers Private Limited.
A - 12, Second Floor, Sector - 2,
Noida - 201 301,
Uttar Pradesh, India, +911204556600
Email: customerservice@thieme.in
www.thieme.in

Cover design: © Thieme
Cover image source: © Thieme
Typesetting by RECTO Graphics, India

Printed in India

5 4 3 2 1

DOI: 10.1055/b000000955

ISBN: 978-93-95390-84-2
Also available as an e-book:
eISBN (PDF): 978-93-95390-85-9
eISBN (epub): 978-93-95390-87-3

Important note: Medicine is an ever-changing science undergoing continual development. Research and clinical experience are continually expanding our knowledge, in particular, our knowledge of proper treatment and drug therapy. Insofar as this book mentions any dosage or application, readers may rest assured that the authors, editors, and publishers have made every effort to ensure that such references are in accordance with **the state of knowledge at the time of production of the book**.

Nevertheless, this does not involve, imply, or express any guarantee or responsibility on the part of the publishers in respect to any dosage instructions and forms of applications stated in the book. **Every user is requested to examine carefully** the manufacturers' leaflets accompanying each drug and to check, if necessary, in consultation with a physician or specialist, whether the dosage schedules mentioned therein or the contraindications stated by the manufacturers differ from the statements made in the present book. Such examination is particularly important with drugs that are either rarely used or have been newly released in the market. Every dosage schedule or every form of application used is entirely at the user's own risk and responsibility. The authors and publishers request every user to report to the publishers any discrepancies or inaccuracies noticed. If errors in this work are found after publication, errata will be posted at www.thieme.com on the product description page.

Some of the product names, patents, and registered designs referred to in this book are in fact registered trademarks or proprietary names even though specific reference to this fact is not always made in the text. Therefore, the appearance of a name without designation as proprietary is not to be construed as a representation by the publisher that it is in the public domain.

Thieme addresses people of all gender identities equally. We encourage our authors to use gender-neutral or gender-equal expressions wherever the context allows.

Contents

Foreword

A picture is worth a thousand words.

When this picture is a CT or MRI from Dr. Suri's book the number of words contained in every image increases exponentially.

In 1979 Godfrey N. Hounsfield was awarded the Nobel Prize in Physiology or Medicine for the development of computed assisted tomography. That year I graduated from medical school and since then I have witnessed an incredible evolution in the quality of diagnostic imaging. The application of this imaging revolution to the temporal bone takes us into a new world: the world of "nanoradiology." The author of this book shows images of anatomic structures that we surgeons only see under microscopic vision. The arrows, dots, and stars on the pictures outline details with incredible precision.

The book you have in your hands not only contains beautiful pictures of the imaging of the temporal bone. It also details the anatomical landmarks required for a successful cochlear implantation both in normal and malformed anatomy. The chapters dealing with cochlear malformations summarize the complex classifications currently available, providing a beautiful schematic representation of each malformation along with its respective imaging study. This is a very useful approach to inner ear malformations.

Dr. Neeraj Suri has to be complimented for putting together an excellent "clear text–beautiful imaging" book on temporal bone landmarks for cochlear implantation, providing a complete three-dimensional understanding of the cochlea and surrounding structures. The author has to be commended for this fine contribution to the literature in the field of cochlear implantation.

I strongly recommend this book to all surgeons willing to enter into the world of cochlear implants. As you may know, cochlear implant surgery is usually simple and straightforward. But when you crash against a complex case, the operation may become a nightmare. The only way to avoid this nightmare, and its deleterious consequences for the patient, is to have as much information as possible beforehand.

In your hands, you have one of the best information sources to make your future cochlear implants as safe, successful, and uneventful as possible.

Javier Gavilán, MD
Professor and Chairman
Department of Otorhinolaryngology
La Paz University Hospital
Madrid, Spain

Foreword

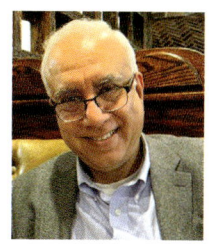

I am honored to write a foreword for this scholarly tome put together by Dr. Neeraj Suri. I consider it an essential reading for the budding otologic and cochlear implant surgeon. A surgeon embarking on a career in this field must be thoroughly conversant and familiar with the radiological features of the temporal bone anatomy. General radiologists or neuroradiologists are generally taught to look for pathology within the temporal bone. They do not however have the luxury of interacting with the patient. Consequently, they are often "flying blind" when it comes to knowing the clinical history, physical examination, and audiological profile of the patient.

From the surgeon's viewpoint it is not only imperative to understand the pathology that exists but also to understand the fine anatomical structures and their spatial relationship to each other. This information is vital in order to generate a mental roadmap in order to execute a successful operation and to achieve optimal results for the patient. Hence, it is vitally important for the surgeon to force himself or herself to delve into the depths of understanding the cross-sectional anatomy of the temporal bone by reading CT scans and MRI scans themselves. Reviewing imaging studies before, during, and following a surgical operation is vitally important in learning pattern recognition and building your own confidence to execute a successful operation with flawless results.

I found the chapters succinct, easy to read, and generously embellished with high-quality images. These are in my view the highlight of Dr Suri's efforts. I would suggest that the reader read, assimilate, and internalize the information and then use the book as a reference tool when rare congenital anomalies are encountered in one's own clinical practice. Chapters on salvaging the infected implant and taking care of patients with hemophilia are particularly engaging.

The chapters in this book are very well organized, easy to read and comprehend, and are copiously illustrated. It is clearly a labor of love in order to promote learning, understanding, and educating the younger group of cochlear implant surgeons. I compliment and thank Dr Suri for doing the hard work. India and the world need more of you. Congratulations Dr. Neeraj Suri!

I wish the book all success.

Arun K. Gadre, MD, FACS, MS, (Bom) DORL
Clinical Professor of Otology, Neurotology and
Skull Base Surgery
Department of Otolaryngology–Head & Neck Surgery;
Director of Otology & Neurotology
Geisinger Commonwealth School of Medicine
Geisinger Medical Center
Danville, Pennsylvania, USA

Preface

In the pursuit of enhancing knowledge in the field of cochlear implantation, it gives me immense pleasure to pen down a book on *Imaging Handbook on Anatomy of Cochlea*. Permit me to give you a little background detail. Over the years, I have faced various difficulties during cochlear implant surgery. At that point of time, I realized that I may have learnt all the tips and tricks of the surgery of cochlear implant but not the imaging.

The difference between a successful and good surgeon is knowing your patient completely. This accelerated my curiosity in all operated cases. With every imaging, I have learnt something new. This book would encourage young surgeon to scrutinize well and make efficacious decisions. It is to sensitize them what we have to look for in the imaging. I feel imaging is a wonderful world provided you learn to understand it.

It is my belief that ideal opinion in cochlear implant can only be obtained when realistic picture is given to the family especially in case of malformations.

As I pen down the preface of this book, I am filled with a profound sense of gratitude and admiration for many individuals who have been instrumental in shaping the trajectory of my journey in the field of cochlear implants, my mentors—Professor Dr. Shankar Medikeri, Bangalore and Professor Dr. Narayanan Janakiram, Trichy, India.

The kind words of advice from Dr. Arun Gadre and Dr. Javier Gavilán were surely instrumental in encouraging me to achieve more and do better. Dr. Mohan Kameshwaran has been a pillar of support to youngsters like me.

My personal thanks to Dr. Meenesh Juvekar for his expert opinion and friendly collaboration.

My sincere thanks to my cochlear implant fellows—Dr. Rajesh V., Dr. Anshu S., Dr. Vijay P., Dr. Sohini, Dr. Vivekanand, and Dr. Anshul; and my dear residents—Dr. Diva S., Dr. Farhana S., and Dr. Shilpa B for their support.

I hope intended readers will find it useful and help them achieve successful cochlear implant surgeries.

Neeraj Suri, MS (ENT)

1 Computed Tomography/ Magnetic Resonance Imaging: A Surgeon's Perspective

Introduction

- Radiographs give us an overview of the entire temporal bone, indicating the pneumatization of temporal bone.
- They are useful in cochlear implant procedures intraoperatively and postoperatively to evaluate the position and integrity of the cochlear implants.
- The most commonly performed imaging techniques are transorbital view and Stenver's view.
- With evolving technology, many centers are using cone beam computed tomography for postoperative radiography.

High-Resolution Computed Tomography

- It is one of the most important and robust investigations.
- The patient is positioned supine on computed tomography table with no tilt.
- From top of the petrous apex to the inferior tip of the mastoid, axial acquisition is performed with its plane parallel to infraorbitomeatal line.
- Reconstruction is done with overlapping sections in axial, coronal, and sagittal planes of 0.6-mm thickness (**Fig. 1.1**).
- Soft tissue window of about 1-mm thickness is also reconstructed into three-dimensional multiplaner reformats in different planes for better understanding of complex anatomy.

Magnetic Resonance Imaging

- Magnetic resonance imaging (MRI) is performed using 1.5T or 3T MRI unit.
- It is done under sedation for children.
- It is nonintrusive.
- It provides functional information.
- It can visualize anatomy in all the planes (**Fig. 1.2** and **Fig. 1.3**).
- There are different signal intensities for different tissues (**Table 1.1**).

The different contrast images on MRI is depicted in **Flowchart 1.1**.

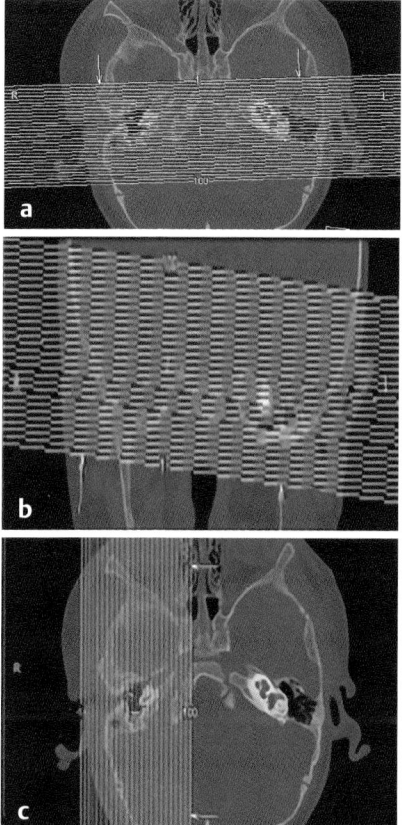

Fig. 1.1 **(a–c)** Scout images of high-resolution computed tomography (HRCT) of temporal bone axial, coronal, and right sagittal sections.

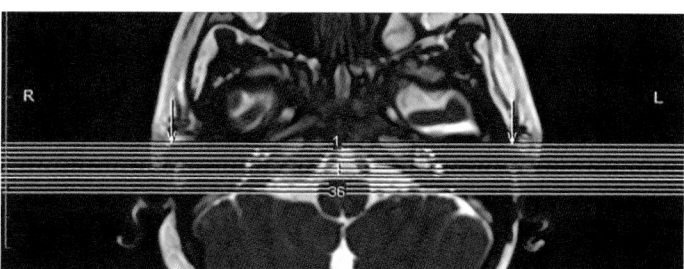

Fig. 1.2 Scout image for magnetic resonance imaging (MRI) scan, axial section.

3

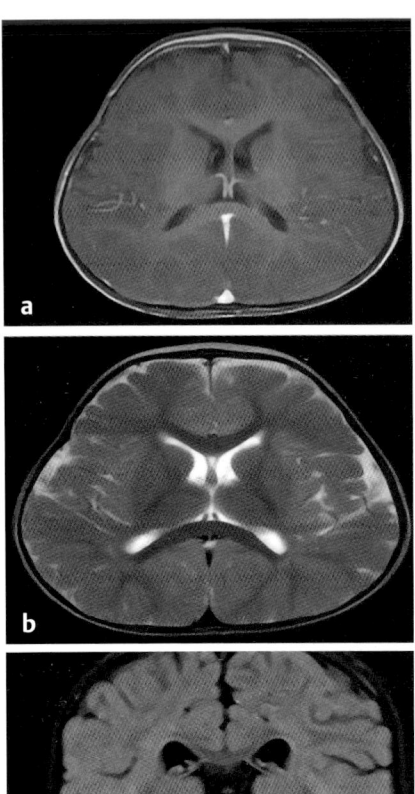

Fig. 1.3 **(a)** Axial T1-weighted image. **(b)** Axial T2-weighted image. **(c)** Coronal T2 fluid-attenuated inversion recovery (FLAIR) image.

Table 1.1 Signal intensity of various tissues on MRI

Tissue	T1-weighted	T2-weighted	FLAIR
CSF	Dark	Bright	Dark
White matter	Light	Dark gray	Dark gray
Cortex	Gray	Light gray	Light gray
Fat	Bright	Light	Light
Inflammation	Dark	Bright	Bright

Abbreviations: CSF, cerebrospinal fluid; FLAIR, fluid-attenuated inversion recovery; MRI, magnetic resonance imaging.

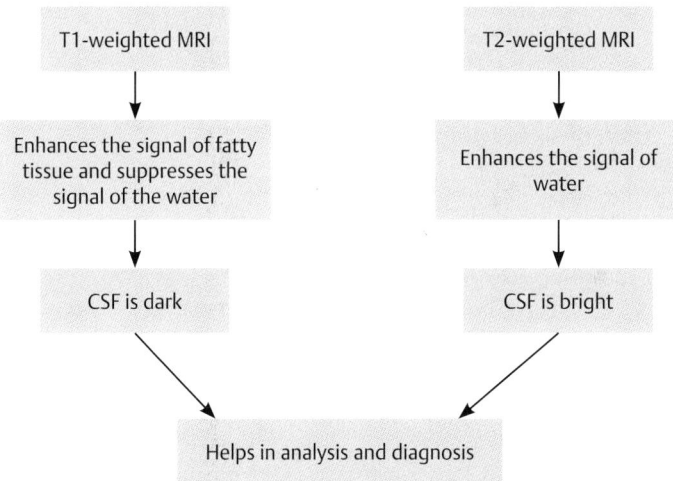

Flowchart 1.1 Difference between T1- and T2-weighted MRI images.

Relative Contraindication of MRI

- Implanted device (magnet needs to be removed in cochlear implant).

Conclusion

- Imaging is a crucial part in the preparation of the cochlear implant candidate as it helps:
  - To identify inner ear structures.
  - To identify congenital and acquired abnormalities.
  - To trace internal auditory canal to facial and cochlear nerve.
  - To differentiate normal from malformed cochlea.
- It helps in anticipation of intraoperative challenges and to prevent complications.

2 Cochlear Implant Related Anatomy: Temporal Bone

Introduction

A cochlear implant surgeon should have a thorough understanding of the intricate anatomy of the temporal bone. Possessing knowledge of the three-dimensional orientation of various structures and their inter-relationships helps in identifying intraoperative surgical landmarks while performing cochlear implant surgeries. It also helps to plan a rational surgical approach, especially in cases with middle ear as well as inner ear anomalies or abnormalities.

External Ear

The external ear has two parts, namely, the pinna and external auditory canal.

Tympanic Membrane

- It is 10 mm in diameter and attaches to the tympanic annulus (**Fig. 2.1**).

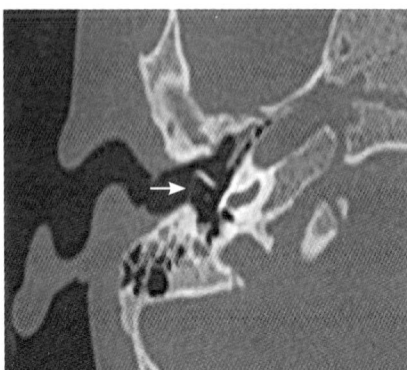

Fig. 2.1 Axial high-resolution computed tomography (HRCT) of temporal bone showing tympanic membrane (*white arrow*).

- It is faintly discerned on computed tomography (CT) images.
- Lateral one-third is fibrocartilaginous.
- Medial two-thirds is surrounded by the tympanic part of temporal bone.

Middle Ear

- It is an air-filled cavity within the petrous portion of the temporal bone.
- It contains an ossicular channel which is bounded by the following:
    - Laterally by tympanic membrane.
    - Medially by inner ear structure.
    - Superiorly by tegmen.
    - Inferiorly by jugular bulb.
- Scutum: A sharp bony projection to which the tympanic membrane is attached superiorly (**Fig. 2.2**).
- Tegmen: It is a thin plate of bone separating middle cranial fossa from the mastoid cavity (**Fig. 2.3**).

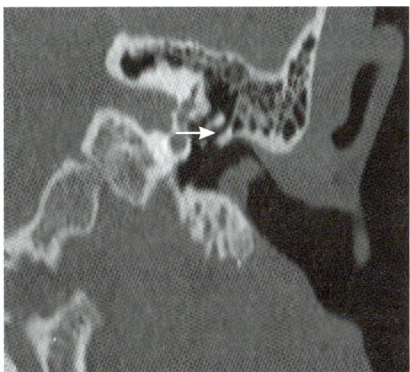

Fig. 2.2 High-resolution computed tomography (HRCT) of temporal bone coronal section showing scutum (*white arrow*).

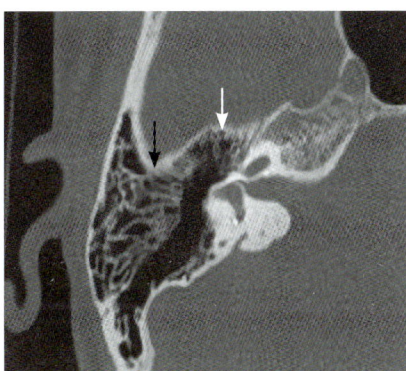

Fig. 2.3 High-resolution computed tomography (HRCT) of temporal bone axial section showing tegmen tympani (*white arrow*) and tegmen mastoideum (*black arrow*).

- Roof of the middle ear cavity is formed by the tegmen tympani.
- Roof of the mastoid cavity is formed by the tegmen mastoideum.
- Posterior wall is formed by the facial recess also known as facial nerve recess. Pyramidal eminence overlies the stapedius muscle.
- Subiculum separates the sinus tympani from the round window niche.

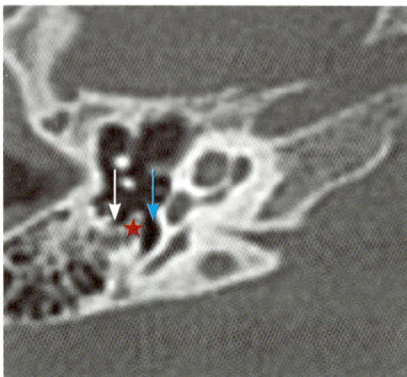

Fig. 2.4 High-resolution computed tomography (HRCT) of temporal bone axial section showing pyramidal eminence (*red star*), sinus tympani (*blue arrow*), and facial recess (*white arrow*).

- Lateral to the pyramidal eminence is the facial recess where lies the second genu of the facial nerve.
- The facial recess is used by the surgeon to place cochlear implant electrode via round window (**Fig. 2.4**).
- Prussak's space also known as superior recess is bounded by the following:
  - Laterally by pars flaccida, scutum.
  - Superiorly by lateral malleal ligament.
  - Medially by neck of malleus.
- Middle ear is subdivided into:
  - Epitympanum.
  - Mesotympanum.
  - Hypotympanum (opening of eustachian tube, internal carotid artery along its medial margin) (**Fig. 2.5**).
- Mesotympanum consists of ossicular chain.
  - Malleus—head, neck, anterior process, lateral process, and manubrium.
  - Incus—body, short process, long process, lenticular process.
  - Stapes—head, anterior crus, posterior crus, foot plate.

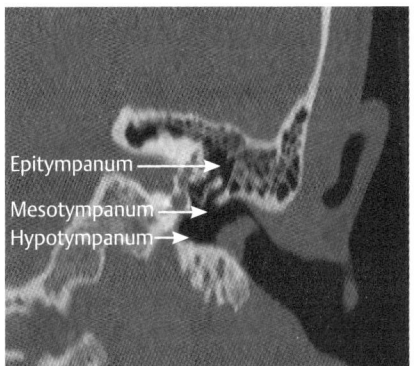

Fig. 2.5 Subdivisions of the middle ear.

- The manubrium of the malleus is attached to the tympanic membrane, and the head of the malleus articulates with the body of the incus in the epi-tympanum forming incudomalleal joint (ice-cream cone appearance which is seen in axial section of high-resolution computed tomography [HRCT] of temporal bone).
- The neck of the malleus anteriorly and the long process of the incus posteriorly give "two dots" appearance.
- The manubrium of the malleus anteriorly and the long process of the incus posteriorly are seen as two parallel lines.
- The lenticular process of the incus extends approximately at right angle from the long process of the incus.
- The head of the stapes and the long process of the incus articulate together to form the incudostapedial joint.
- The foot plate of the stapes attaches to the oval window of the vestibule.
- There are four suspensory ossicular ligaments:
  - Superior malleal.
  - Lateral malleal.

11

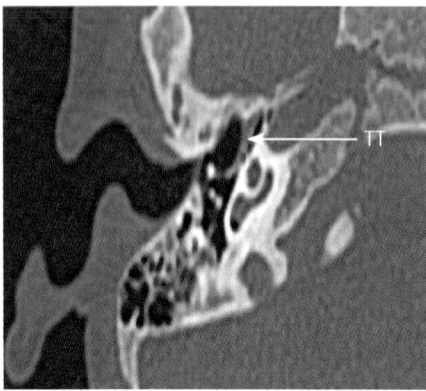

Fig. 2.6 High-resolution computed tomography (HRCT) of temporal bone axial section showing tensor tympani (TT) muscle.

- Posterior malleal.
- Posterior incudal.

- The suspensory ossicular ligaments are seen on CT image as thin linear structures.
- The lateral malleal ligament is the most commonly identified ligament among all suspensory ligaments.
- The tensor tympani muscle arises from the cartilaginous part of the eustachian tube, and then turns sharply at cochleariformis process and attaches to the neck of the malleus (**Fig. 2.6**).
- Epitympanum communicates with the mastoid via the aditus and antrum.
- Mastoid is an air-filled cavity:
  - It is divided into numerous compartments by mastoid septations (**Fig. 2.7**).
  - Air cell sizes are variable.

- Korner's septum: It is a bony structure (petrosquamous suture) separating mastoid air cells into two compartments. When thick may be confused with medial wall of the antrum by the surgeon.

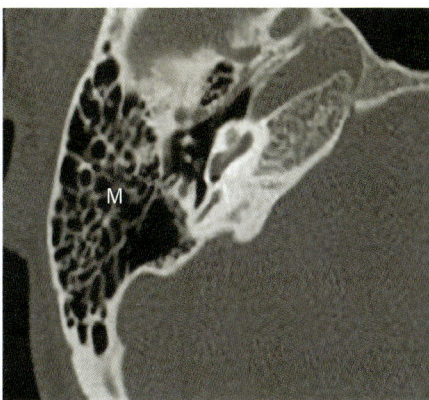

Fig. 2.7 High-resolution computed tomography (HRCT) of temporal bone axial section showing pneumatized mastoid (M) bone.

- Petromastoid canal is a channel passing between superior and lateral semicircular canal.
  - Commuting cranial cavity to mastoid antrum.
  - Measures 0.5 to 1 mm.
  - Contains subarcuate artery.
  - Potential channel for spread of infection to and from the mastoid antrum.
  - Not to be mistaken for fracture line.

Inner Ear

- It is situated in petrous part of temporal bone.
- It comprises bony and membranous labyrinth.

Cochlea

- It is a snail-like structure.
- It consists of basal turn, middle turn, and apical turn, which are separated by interscalar septae (**Fig. 2.8a–c**).

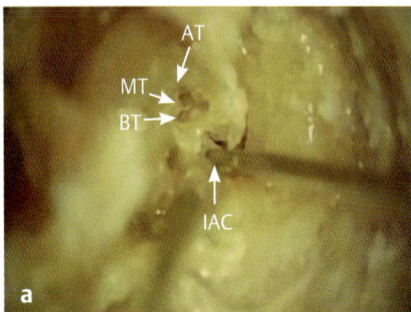

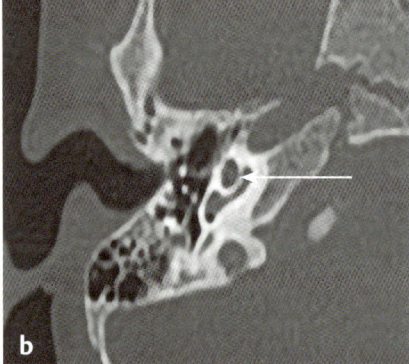

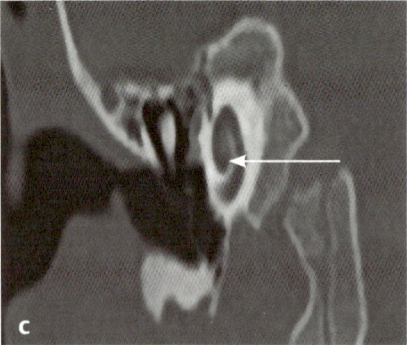

Fig. 2.8 **(a)** Apical turn (AT), middle turn (MT), basal turn (BT), and internal auditory canal (IAC). **(b)** Axial high-resolution computed tomography (HRCT) of temporal bone showing apical, middle, and basal turn of cochlea (*white arrow*). **(c)** Coronal HRCT of temporal bone showing cochlea with its turns (*white arrow*).

- The osseous spiral lamina is well appreciated on T2 magnetic resonance imaging (MRI). It parallels the interscalar septae.

Cochlear Promontory

- The bulge of cochlear promontory is prominently seen in the middle ear cavity as a dome (**Fig. 2.9**).
- Nerve of Jacobson courses above the promontory.
- Vestibule is ovoid shape, located superior and posterior to the cochlea.

Semicircular Canals

- They are three in number:
    - Superior.
    - Posterior.
    - Lateral semicircular canal.
- They are placed at right angle to each other.
- Each has ampulla at one end.
- Posterior and superior semicircular canals have a common crus.

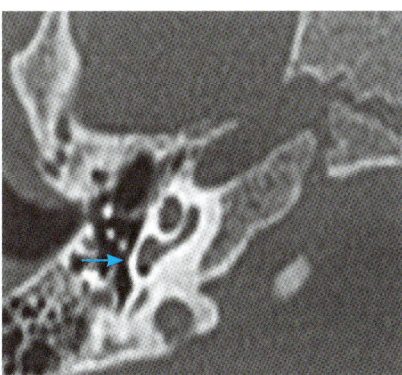

Fig. 2.9 High-resolution computed tomography (HRCT) of temporal bone axial section showing cochlear promontory (*blue arrow*).

- The lateral semicircular canal has two separate openings into the vestibule (**Fig. 2.10a, b**).
- The endolymphatic duct runs from the vestibule and ends in a blind pouch in the posterior cranial fossa.
- Vestibular aqueduct:
  - Envelopes endolymphatic duct.
  - 1 mm at mid-point and 2 mm at operculum.

- Cochlear aqueduct is a narrow bony channel that surrounds perilymphatic duct and extends from the basal turn of the cochlea anterior (round window) to the subarachnoid space.
  - It measures 0.1 to 0.2 mm in the midportion.

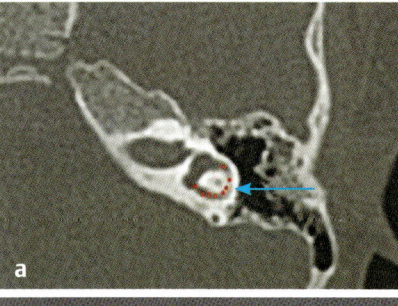

Fig. 2.10 (**a**) High-resolution computed tomography (HRCT) axial section showing lateral semicircular canal (*red dots and blue arrow*). (**b**) HRCT coronal section showing superior (S-SCC) and lateral (L-SCC) semicircular canals.

- It roughly runs parallel and immediately inferior to the internal auditory canal (approximately 6–7 mm).

- Internal auditory canal:
  - It runs in petrous bone.
  - It has porus acousticus at its medial end and labyrinth at the lateral end.
  - Transverse crest (crista falciformis) divides the internal auditory canal into two compartments (superior and inferior) (**Fig. 2.11**).

- The facial nerve along with superior vestibular nerve runs in the superior compartment and the cochlear nerve with inferior vestibular nerve runs in the inferior compartment (**Fig. 2.12**).

- Superior and inferior vestibular nerves run in superior–posterior and inferior–posterior compartments.

Mnemonic: Seven Up Coke Down—Facial nerve (7th nerve) up and cochlea down

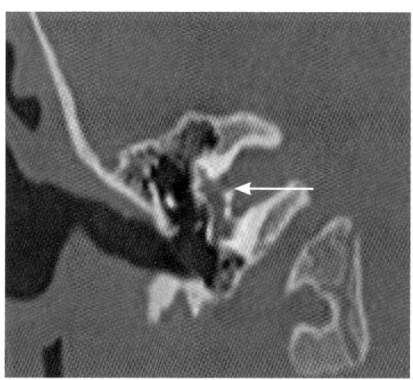

Fig. 2.11 High-resolution computed tomography (HRCT) of temporal bone coronal section showing falciform crest (*white arrow*).

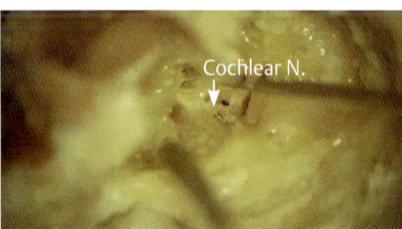

Fig. 2.12 Cochlear nerve.

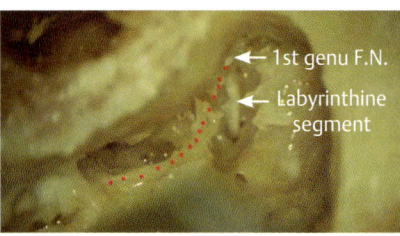

Fig. 2.13 Labyrinthine segment and the first genu of the facial nerve.

Facial Nerve

- Its bony canal defines its course in HRCT images.
- It is divided into three segments—labyrinthine, tympanic, and mastoid.
- Labyrinthine segment begins at the fundus of the internal auditory canal and courses anteriorly ending at the geniculate ganglion (**Fig. 2.13**). It runs between the vestibule and cochlea.
- The first genu takes hair-pin turn and extends posteriorly as the tympanic segment. Here it gives rise to the greater superficial petrosal nerve (**Fig. 2.13**).

On Coronal CT Images

- The tympanic segment and the labyrinthine segment of the facial nerve can be visualized as snake eyes.
- It runs inferior to the lateral semicircular canal and superolateral to the oval window (**Fig. 2.14**).

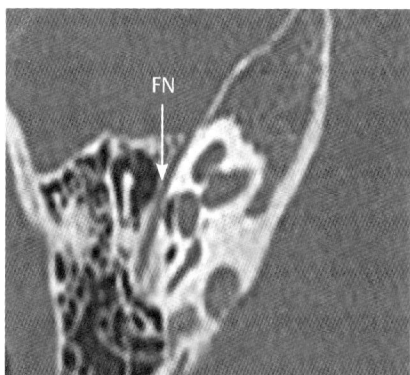

Fig. 2.14 High-resolution computed tomography (HRCT) of temporal bone axial section showing the tympanic segment of the facial nerve (FN) canal.

- The second genu is between the facial recess laterally and the pyramidal eminence medially.
- The tympanic segment of the facial nerve runs inferior to the short process of the incus and turns at the genu to become the mastoid segment.
- Mastoid segment:
    - It courses vertically to exit through the stylomastoid foramen.
    - It gives the stapedius nerve and chorda tympani nerve (runs into the middle ear cavity).
    - Singular nerve supplies the ampulla of the posterior semicircular canal.

If the tympanic segment is dehiscent, the surgeon needs to be extra careful to avoid facial palsy.

3 Radiology of Normal Cochlea

Introduction

There has been an enormous increase in the number of cochlear implant surgeries over the past decade. This in turn has led to an increase in the preoperative imaging process done before the surgical procedure. The baseline investigations include high-resolution computed tomography (HRCT) and magnetic resonance imaging (MRI) of the temporal bones, which are crucial to provide vital information. However, MRI is now increasingly being used to study the membranous labyrinth and the cranial nerves; it provides accurate information about fine details of the anatomical structures.

Axial HRCT Images of Temporal Bone

Fig. 3.1, Fig. 3.2, Fig. 3.3, Fig. 3.4, Fig. 3.5, Fig. 3.6, Fig. 3.7, Fig. 3.8, Fig. 3.9, Fig. 3.10, Fig. 3.11, Fig. 3.12, Fig. 3.13, Fig. 3.14, Fig. 3.15, and **Fig. 3.16** show axial scans from upward to down with 0.5 mm cuts.

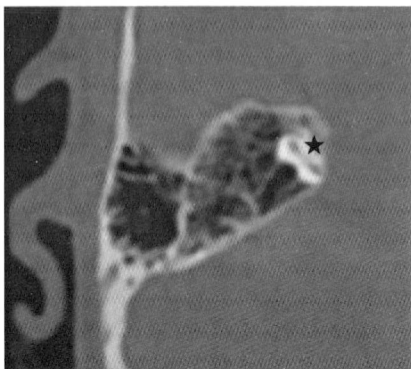

Fig. 3.1 Axial high-resolution computed tomography (HRCT) of temporal bone showing superior semicircular canal (SCC) (*black star*) at petrous apex with pneumatized mastoid air cells.

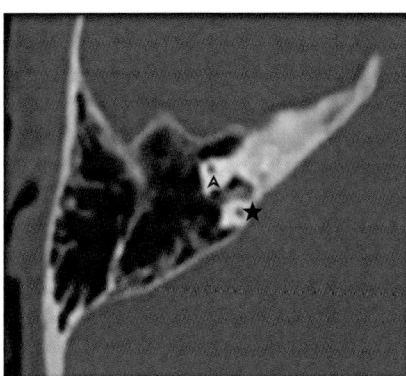

Fig. 3.2 Axial high-resolution computed tomography (HRCT) of temporal bone showing petrous bone consisting of two hollow structures, crus commune (*black star*) and ampulla (*arrowhead*), of superior semicircular canal.

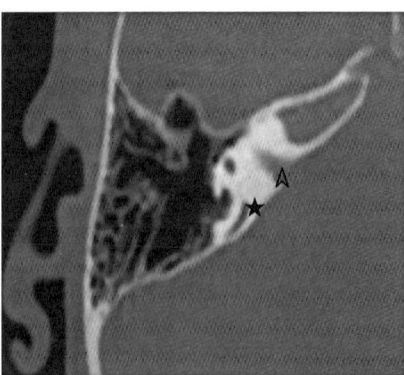

Fig. 3.3 Axial high-resolution computed tomography (HRCT) of temporal bone showing horizontal hollow structure at the site of crus commune, posterior semicircular canal (PSC) (*black star*); beginning of internal auditory canal (*arrowhead*) is seen.

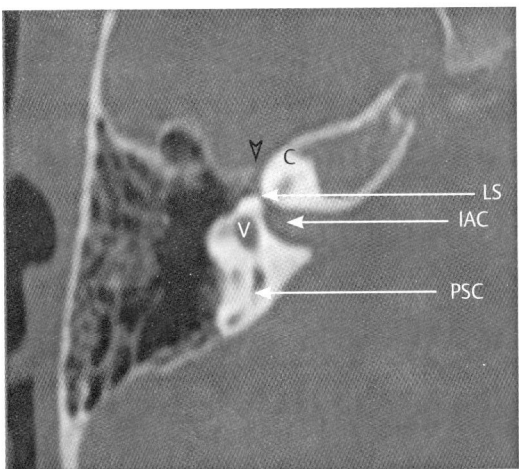

Fig. 3.4 Axial high-resolution computed tomography (HRCT) of temporal bone showing internal auditory canal (IAC), labyrinthine segment of the facial nerve (LS), the first genu of the facial nerve (*arrowhead*), vestibule (V), cochlea (C), and posterior semicircular canal (PSC).

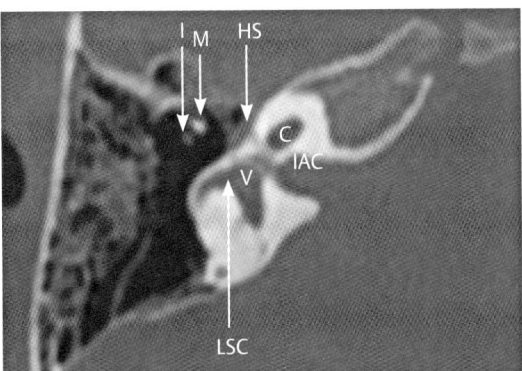

Fig. 3.5 Axial high-resolution computed tomography (HRCT) of temporal bone showing: cochlea (C), internal auditory canal (IAC), vestibule (V), lateral semicircular canal (LSC), malleus head (M), horizontal segment of the facial nerve (HS), and incus (I).

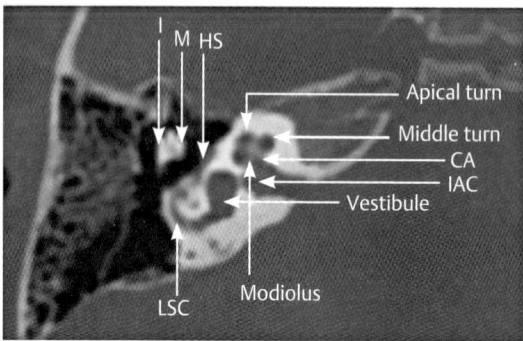

Fig. 3.6 Axial high-resolution computed tomography (HRCT) of temporal bone showing signet ring appearance (LSC), horizontal segment (HS) of the facial nerve bisecting LSC, and head of malleus along with body of incus making classical ice-cream cone appearance. Modiolus is seen (modiolus is whitish structure present in cochlea). CA, cochlear aperture.

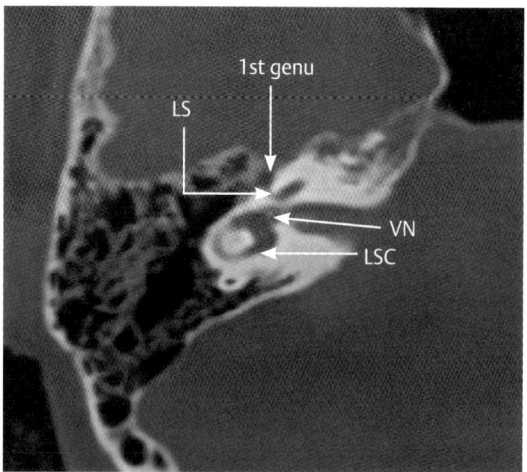

Fig. 3.7 Axial high-resolution computed tomography (HRCT) of temporal bone showing: labyrinthine segment (LS), vestibular nerve (VN), and lateral semicircular canal (LSC).

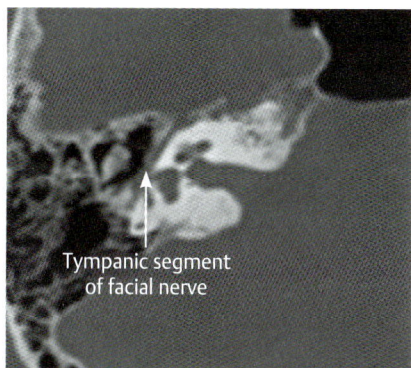

Fig. 3.8 Axial high-resolution computed tomography (HRCT) of temporal bone showing tympanic segment of facial nerve.

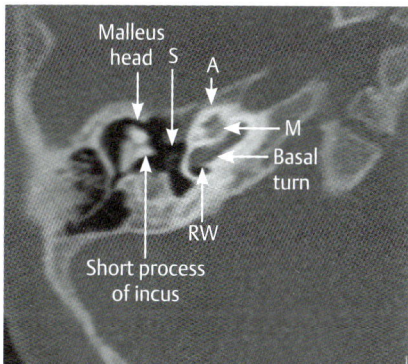

Fig. 3.9 Axial high-resolution computed tomography (HRCT) of temporal bone showing malleus head, basal turn of cochlea, round window (RW), stapes (S), short process of malleus, apical turn of cochlea (A), and middle turn of cochlea (M).

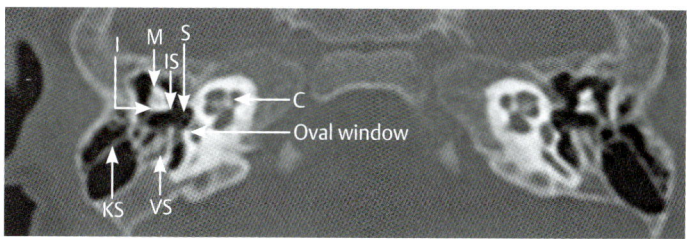

Fig. 3.10 Axial high-resolution computed tomography (HRCT) of temporal bone showing ear ossicles stapes (S), head of malleus (M), body of incus (I), incudostapedial joint (IS), oval window lying below stapes, apical and middle turns of cochlea (C), Korner's septum (KS), and vertical segment of facial nerve (VS).

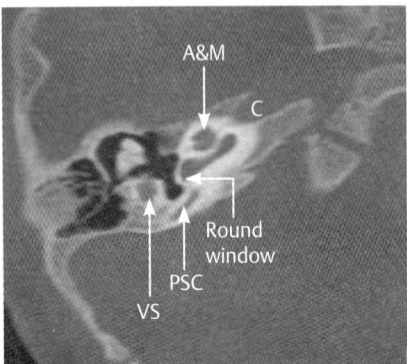

Fig. 3.11 Axial high-resolution computed tomography (HRCT) of temporal bone showing apical and middle turn (A&M), carotid (C), posterior semicircular canal (PSC), vertical segment of facial nerve (VS), and round window (RW).

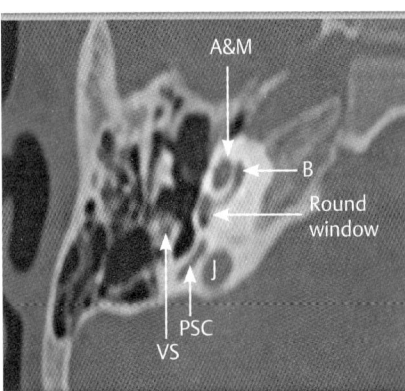

Fig. 3.12 Axial high-resolution computed tomography (HRCT) of temporal bone showing apical and middle turn of cochlea (A&M), basal turn of cochlea (B), round window, vertical segment of facial nerve (VS), posterior semicircular canal (PSC), and jugular bulb (J).

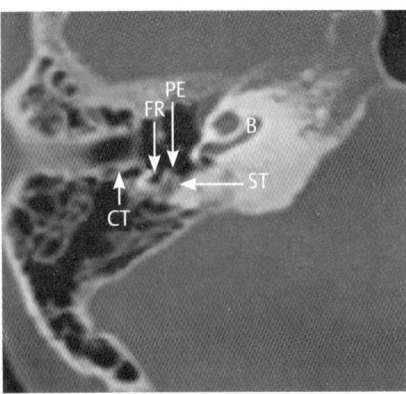

Fig. 3.13 Axial high-resolution computed tomography (HRCT) of temporal bone showing pyramidal eminence (PE), sinus tympani (ST), chorda tympani (CT), facial recess (FR), and basal turn (B). Lateral to pyramidal eminence is facial recess and medial to it is sinus tympani.

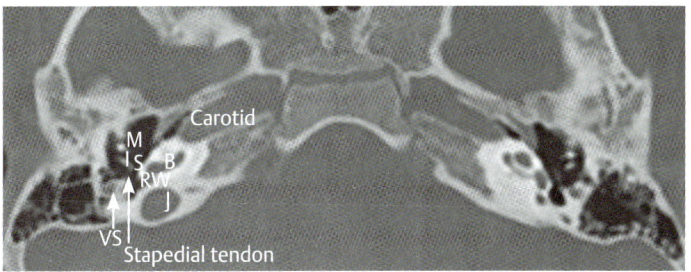

Fig. 3.14 Axial high-resolution computed tomography (HRCT) of temporal bone showing round window (RW), basal turn of cochlea (B), malleus neck (M), incus long process (I), stapes (S) in classical three dot appearance, vertical segment of facial nerve (VS), carotid anteriorly, and jugular bulb (J).

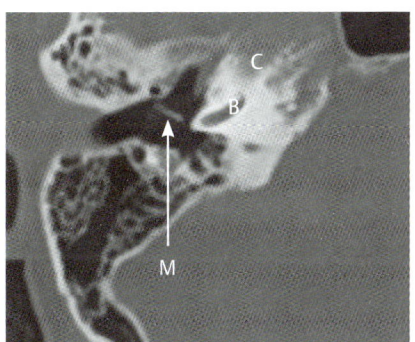

Fig. 3.15 Axial high-resolution computed tomography (HRCT) of temporal bone showing handle of malleus (M), basal turn of cochlea (B), and carotid (C).

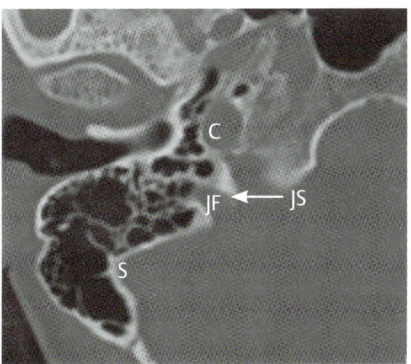

Fig. 3.16 Axial high-resolution computed tomography (HRCT) of temporal bone showing sigmoid (S), carotid canal (C), jugular spine (JS), and jugular foramen (JF).

Posterior semicircular canal is seen running parallel to petrous apex.

- Cochlear structures are always anterior to the internal auditory canal (IAC) and vestibular structures are posterior to the IAC.

Fig. 3.17, Fig. 3.18, Fig. 3.19, Fig. 3.20, Fig. 3.21, Fig. 3.22, Fig. 3.23, Fig. 3.24, Fig. 3.25, Fig. 3.26, and **Fig. 3.27** show coronal HRCT images of temporal bone.

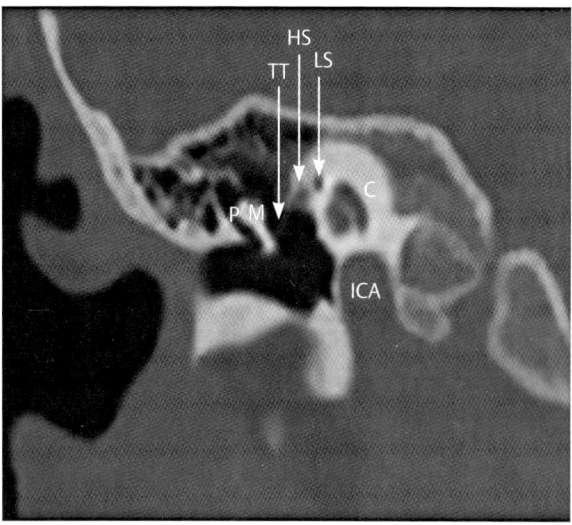

Fig. 3.17 Coronal high-resolution computed tomography (HRCT) of temporal bone showing (from anterior to posterior) pneumatized mastoid air cells, Prussak's space (P), lateral to head of malleus (M), horizontal segment (HS) of facial nerve laterally, and labyrinthine segment (LS) of facial nerve medially lying above cochlea (C) forming classical snail eye appearance. A faint gray structure from malleus going upward is tensor tympani tendon (TT). ICA, internal carotid artery.

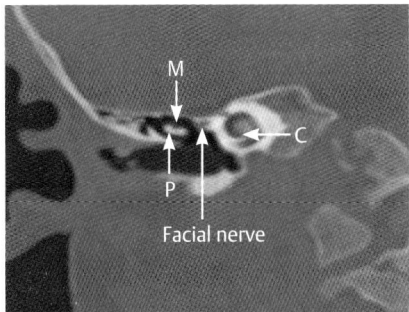

Fig. 3.18 Coronal high-resolution computed tomography (HRCT) of temporal bone showing cochlea (C), Prussak's space (P), malleus (M), and facial nerve.

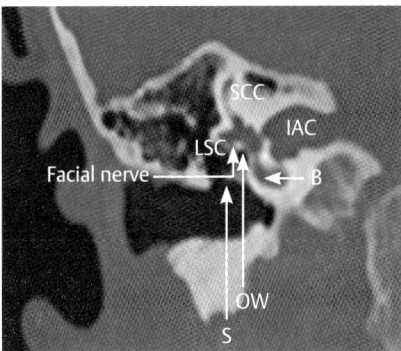

Fig. 3.19 Coronal high-resolution computed tomography (HRCT) of temporal bone showing headless mermaid appearance by superior semicircular canal (SCC), lateral semicircular canal (LSC), internal auditory canal (IAC), facial nerve, oval window opening (OW) with stapes (S), and basal turn of cochlea in coronal section (B).

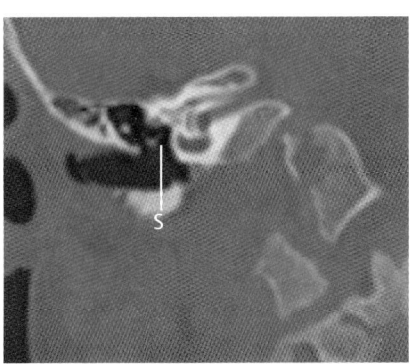

Fig. 3.20 Coronal high-resolution computed tomography (HRCT) of temporal bone showing stapes (S).

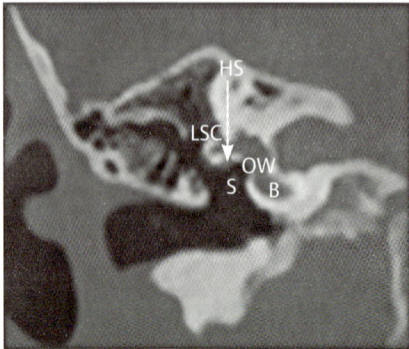

Fig. 3.21 Coronal high-resolution computed tomography (HRCT) of temporal bone showing lateral semicircular canal (LSC) above horizontal segment (HS) of facial nerve, oval window (OW), basal turn (B), and stapes (S).

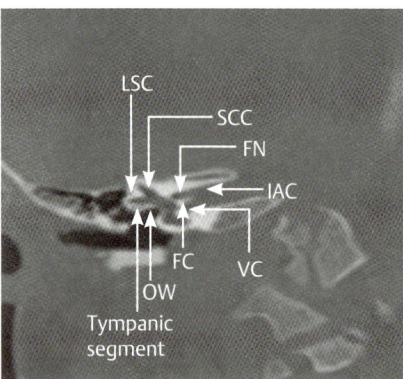

Fig. 3.22 Coronal high-resolution computed tomography (HRCT) of temporal bone showing lateral semicircular canal (LSC), superior semicircular canal (SCC), facial nerve (FN), internal auditory canal (IAC), vestibulocochlear nerve (VC), oval window (OW), falciform crest (FC), and tympanic segment of facial nerve.

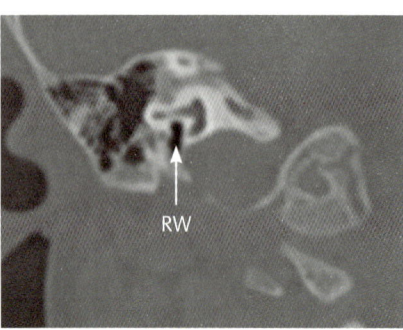

Fig. 3.23 Coronal high-resolution computed tomography (HRCT) of temporal bone showing round window (RW).

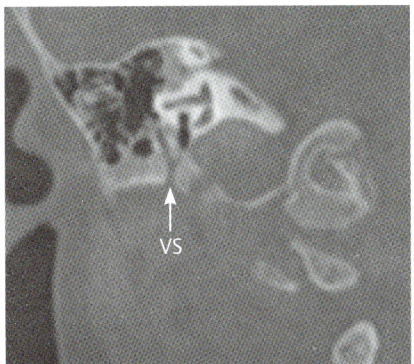

Fig. 3.24 Coronal high-resolution computed tomography (HRCT) of temporal bone showing vertical segment of facial nerve (VS).

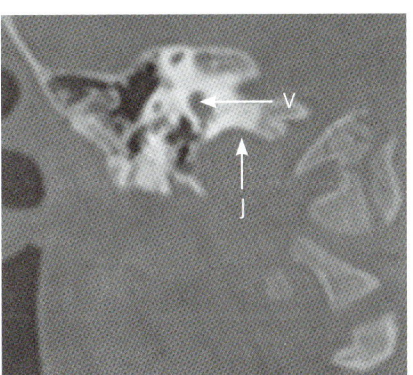

Fig. 3.25 Coronal high-resolution computed tomography (HRCT) of temporal bone showing vestibule (V) and jugular bulb (J).

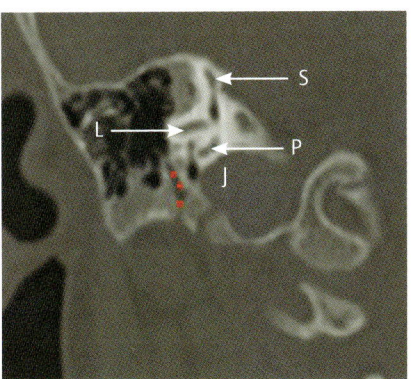

Fig. 3.26 Coronal high-resolution computed tomography (HRCT) of temporal bone showing lateral semicircular canal (L), posterior semicircular canal (P), superior semicircular canal (S), and jugular bulb (J). *Red dots* show vertical segment of facial nerve.

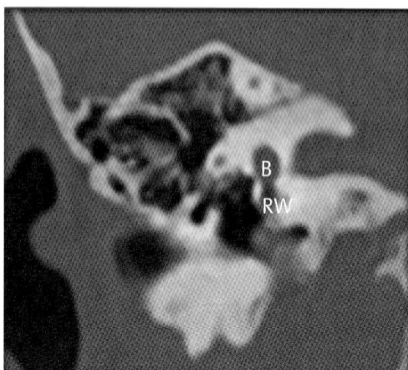

Fig. 3.27 Coronal high-resolution computed tomography (HRCT) of temporal bone showing basal turn of cochlea (B) and round window (RW) opening.

Magnetic Resonance Imaging of the Temporal Bone

Magnetic resonance imaging (MRI) is used for diagnostic purpose in temporal bone. It enhances soft tissue whereas CT scan gives detailed picture of bony structures.

- For cochlear implants in particular, we use T2 images because the white contrast of the fluid helps visualize inner ear and nerves in contrast (**Fig. 3.28, Fig. 3.29, Fig. 3.30, Fig. 3.31, Fig. 3.32, Fig. 3.33, Fig. 3.34,** and **Fig. 3.35**).
- MRI is done to:
    - Visualize fluid-containing spaces of temporal bone, (i.e., inner ear).
    - Evaluate the 7th and 8th nerve complex.
    - Assess ossification/patency of cochlea.
    - Detect lesion in cerebellopontine angle (CPA)/petrous apex.
    - Detect gliotic (damaged area in brain) areas, especially in Wernicke's and Broca's area.

Note: Hypoxic injury during birth is a prominent risk factor for hearing loss in children. In such cases hyperintensity is noted in periventricular area. Hypoglycemic injury is visualized as hyperintensity in periorbital area.

As a rule, Broca's area controls dexterity. In 90% of cases Broca's area is functional in left side post basal frontal area because right-handed individuals are far more common than left.

T2 MRI Axial Cuts—From Superior to Inferior

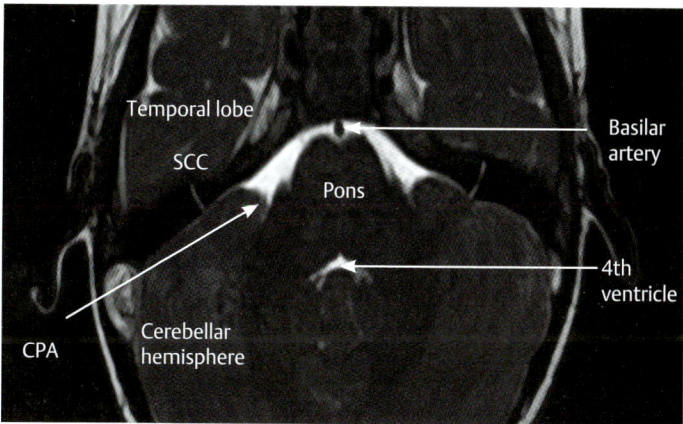

Fig. 3.28 T2 magnetic resonance imaging (MRI) showing superior semicircular canal (SCC) as gray slit-like structure, temporal lobe anteriorly, cerebellar hemisphere posteriorly, and pons and cerebellopontine angle (CPA) medially.

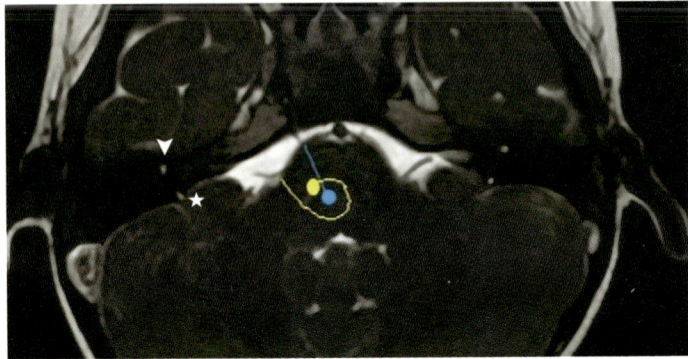

Fig. 3.29 T2 magnetic resonance imaging (MRI) showing crus commune (*white star*) and ampulla of superior semicircular canal (*arrowhead*). For better understanding, approximate position of nucleus of abducens nerve (*blue dot*) with the nerve which is continuing in black and nucleus for facial nerve (*yellow dot*) with the nerve circling nucleus of abducent finally emerging out of cerebellopontine angle (CPA) has been drawn.

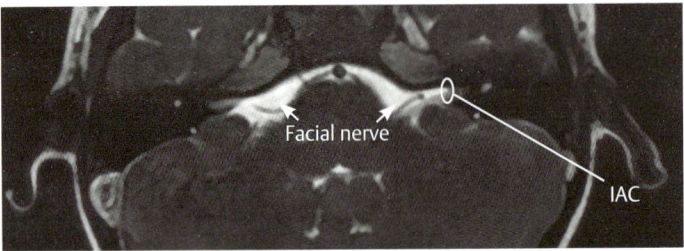

Fig. 3.30 T2 magnetic resonance imaging (MRI) axial section showing facial nerve emerging from pons to internal auditory canal (IAC) via cerebellopontine angle. The oval mark indicates the IAC.

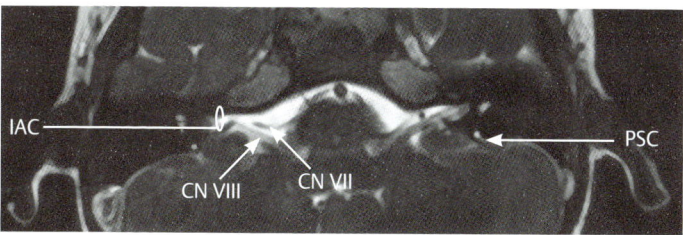

Fig. 3.31 Cranial nerve (CN) VIII (vestibulocochlear) and CN VII (facial) emerging from cerebellopontine angle and entering to internal auditory canal (IAC); posterior semicircular canal (PSC) is seen from crus commune.

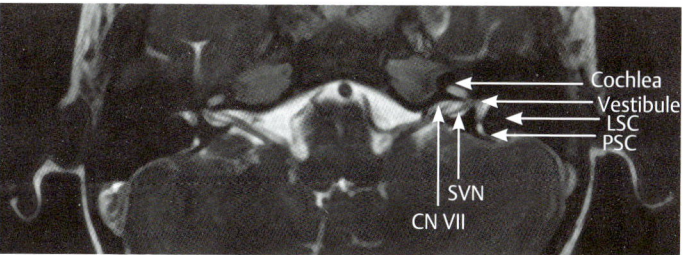

Fig. 3.32 Image showing the middle turn of cochlea, vestibule, posterior semicircular canal (PSC), and lateral semicircular canal (LSC). In the internal auditory canal (IAC), the facial nerve lies anteriorly and superiorly while the superior vestibular nerve (SVN) lies posteriorly to it.

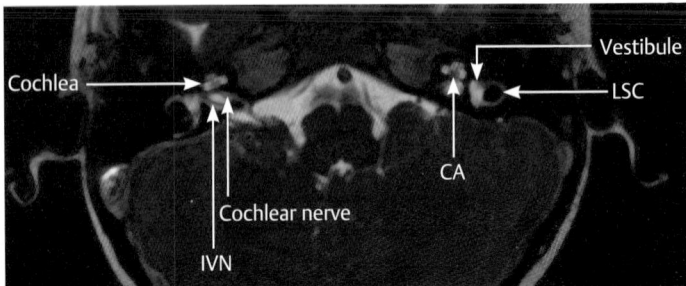

Fig. 3.33 Image showing apical and middle turn of cochlea, cochlear nerve and inferior vestibular nerve (IVN) in internal auditory canal (IAC), lateral semicircular canal (LSC), vestibule, and cochlear aperture (CA) where cochlear nerve enters into cochlea.

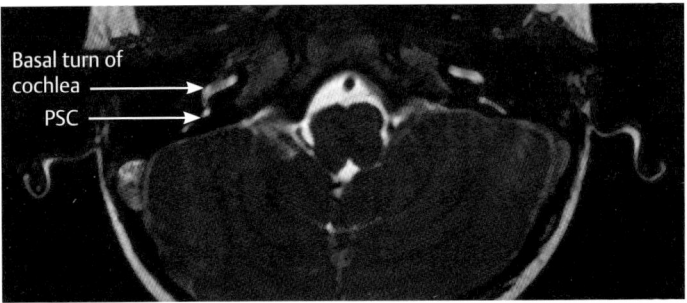

Fig. 3.34 Basal turn of cochlea and posterior semicircular canal (PSC). Note cochlea is filled with fluid; hence, it is white in T2 image. In case of ossification this contrast is visibly reduced.

Sagittal T2 MRI Images

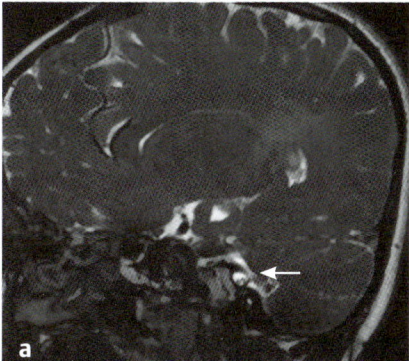

Fig. 3.35 **(a–c)** Sagittal T2 magnetic resonance imaging (MRI). The *arrow* is showing a bunch of nerves exiting cerebellopontine junction into internal auditory meatus. Inferior vestibular nerve (IVN) and superior vestibular nerve (SVN).

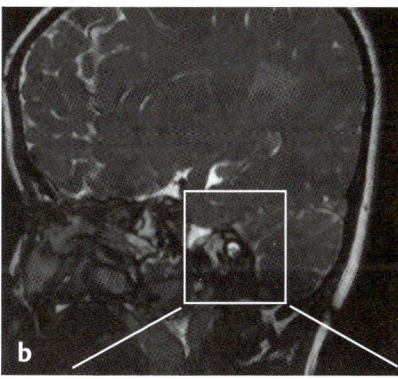

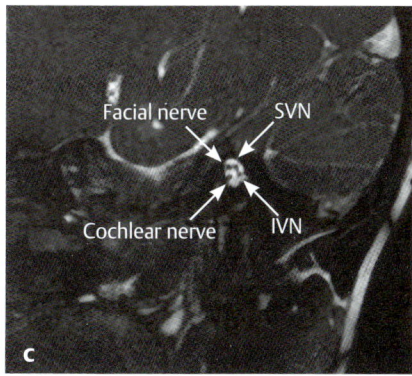

4 Facial Nerve in Cochlear Implants

Introduction

The total length of the facial nerve is 30 mm. It has five segments, namely, intracranial, intracanalicular, labyrinthine, tympanic, and mastoid. The facial nerve exits the brainstem from ponto-medullary junction and enters the internal auditory canal (IAC) along with cranial nerve VIII. The diameter of meatal foramen from where the nerve exits the canal is 0.68 mm, which is the narrowest part of the nerve.

- Intimate knowledge of the relevant surgical anatomy of facial recess is important to safely perform the posterior tympanotomy.
- Facial recess is a triangular space defined medially by the mastoid segment of the facial nerve, laterally by the chorda tympani nerve, and superiorly by the incudal fossa.
- The complication of the facial nerve palsy generally occurs because of the limited understanding of the anatomy of the facial recess and different types of facial nerve anomalies.
- It is observed that inner ear malformation and cochlear hypoplasia are associated with facial anomalies.

Morphology of the Facial Nerve

Morphology of the facial nerve is divided into meatal segment, labyrinthine segment, tympanic segment, and mastoid segment.

- Meatal segment is in the IAC.
- Labyrinthine segment starts from the anterior superior part of the fundus of IAC and extends up to the first genu (**Fig. 4.1** and **Fig. 4.2**).
- Tympanic segment is evaluated according to the important landmark (oval window and lateral

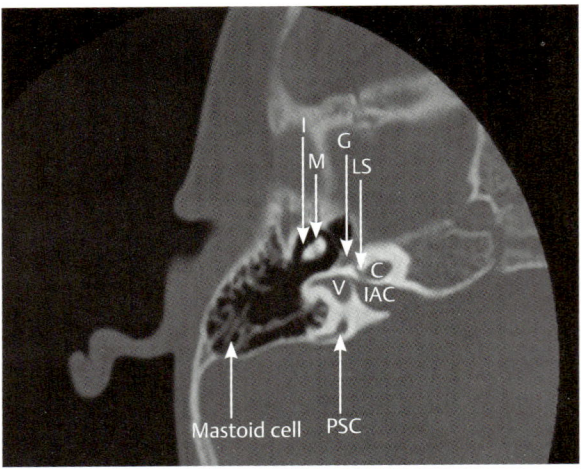

Fig. 4.1 Axial high-resolution computed tomography (HRCT) of temporal bone showing well-pneumatized mastoid air cells. Geniculate ganglion (1st genu of facial nerve) (G), posterior semicircular canal (PSC), vestibule (V), malleus (M), incus (I), middle turn of cochlea (C), internal auditory canal (IAC), and labyrinthine segment (LS) of the facial nerve appeared in the section arising from the IAC.

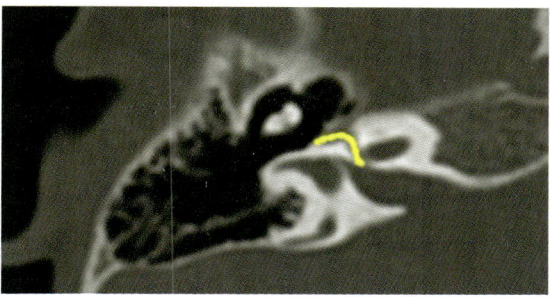

Fig. 4.2 Axial high-resolution computed tomography (HRCT) of temporal bone showing zoomed image of previous scan with *yellow mark* showing labyrinthine segment (LS) of the facial nerve arising from the internal auditory canal (IAC), taking a hairpin turn to become the tympanic segment (TS).

semicircular canal). It passes between oval window and lateral semicircular canal.
- Mastoid segment extends from the second genu to the stylomastoid foramen.

According to Sennaroğlu (in 2020), meatal, labyrinthine, tympanic, and mastoid segments are divided into subtypes.

- Meatal segment:
    - Type 1: Normal, >2 mm midpoint of IAC.
    - Type 2: <2 mm, stenotic.
    - Type 3: Bony facial canal.
    - Type 4: Duplication.
- Labyrinthine segment (**Fig. 4.2**):
    - Type 1: Normal.
    - Type 2: Anterior displacement.
    - Type 3: Superior displacement.
    - Type 4: Straight segment.

- Tympanic segment:
  - Type 1: Normal.
  - Type 2: Above oval window.
  - Type 3: At oval window.
  - Type 4: Inferior to oval window.

A normal tympanic segment is superior and lateral to oval window and stapes and inferior to lateral semicircular canal (**Fig. 4.3** and **Fig. 4.4**).

- Mastoid segment:
  - Normally it is difficult to visualize chorda tympani nerve in HRCT so external auditory canal is used for measurements of facial recess (**Fig. 4.5, Fig. 4.6, Fig. 4.7,** and **Fig. 4.8**).
  - Distance between external auditory canal and facial nerve is the width of facial recess:
    - Type 1: >2 mm.
    - Type 2: <2 mm.
    - Type 3: Unclassified.

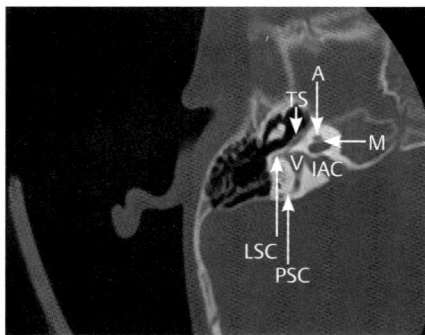

Fig. 4.3 Axial high-resolution computed tomography (HRCT) of temporal bone showing apical (A) and middle (M) turn of cochlea, internal auditory canal (IAC), vestibule (V), lateral semicircular canal (LSC), posterior semicircular canal (PSC), and tympani segment (TS) of the facial nerve.

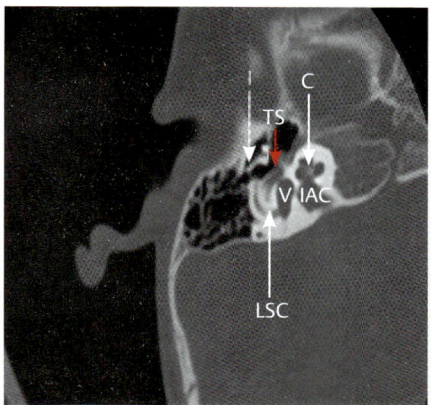

Fig. 4.4 Axial high-resolution computed tomography (HRCT) of temporal bone showing tympanic segment (TS) of facial nerve (*red arrow*) bisecting lateral semicircular canal (LSC), modiolus of cochlea (C), internal auditory canal (IAC), incus (I), vestibule (V), and cochlea.

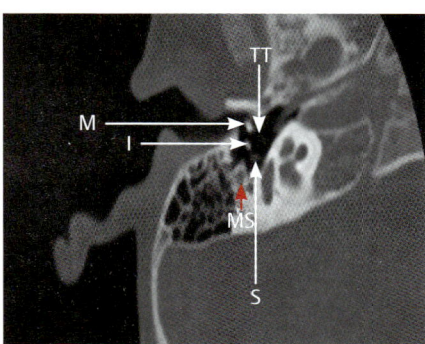

Fig. 4.5 Axial high-resolution computed tomography (HRCT) of temporal bone showing incus (I), malleus (M), stapes (S), tensor tympani (TT), and mastoid segment (MS) of facial nerve (*red arrow*).

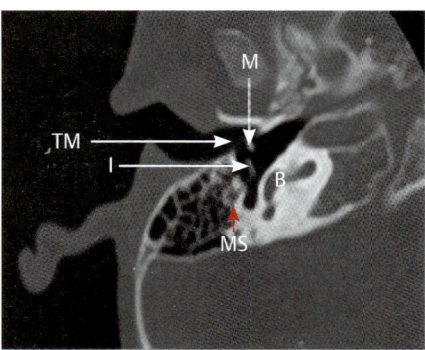

Fig. 4.6 Axial high-resolution computed tomography (HRCT) of temporal bone showing basal turn of cochlea (B), mastoid segment (MS) of facial nerve (*red arrow*) with ear ossicles, tympanic membrane (TM), incus (I), malleus (M).

43

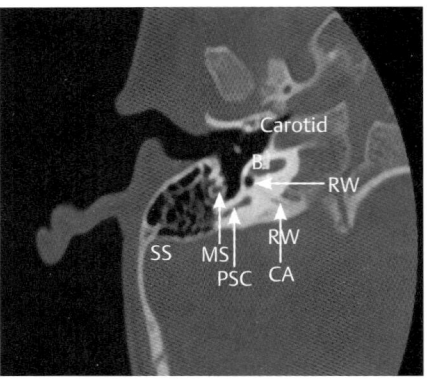

Fig. 4.7 Axial high-resolution computed tomography (HRCT) of temporal bone showing mastoid segment of facial nerve (MS), basal turn of cochlea (B), with round window (RW), cochlear aqueduct (CA), carotid artery, sigmoid sinus (SS), and posterior semicircular canal (PSC).

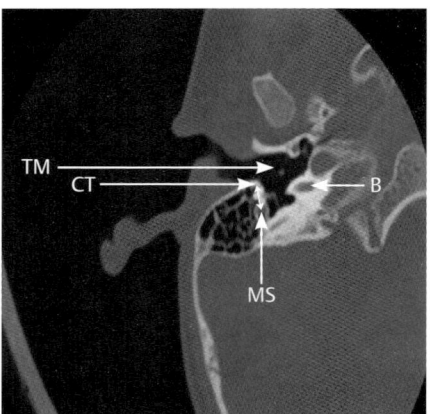

Fig. 4.8 Axial high-resolution computed tomography (HRCT) of temporal bone showing basal turn of cochlea (B), mastoid segment (MS), chorda tympani (CT), and tympanic membrane (TM). Distance between chorda tympani (CT) and mastoid segment (MS) is the width of the facial recess (FR).

Coronal Section of HRCT Scan—Posterior to Anterior

Coronal section of HRCT of temporal bone is presented in **Fig. 4.9, Fig. 4.10, Fig. 4.11,** and **Fig. 4.12**.

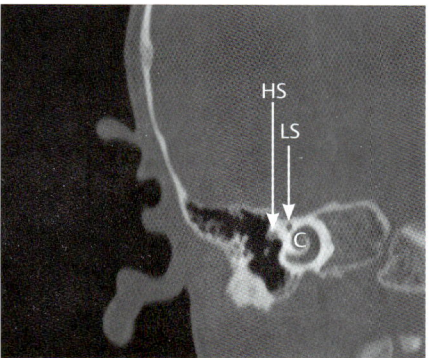

Fig. 4.9 Coronal high-resolution computed tomography (HRCT) of temporal bone showing snake eye appearance of cochlea (C), labyrinthine segment (LS), and tympanic/horizontal segment (HS).

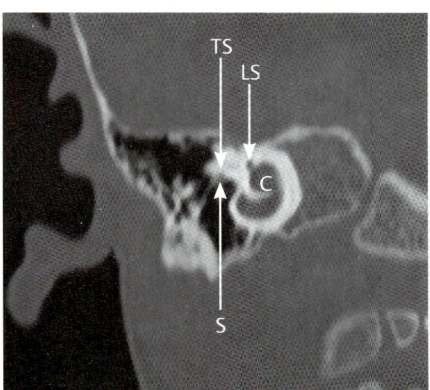

Fig. 4.10 Coronal high-resolution computed tomography (HRCT) of temporal bone showing cochlea (C), stapes (S), labyrinthine segment (LS), and tympanic segment (TS) of facial nerve.

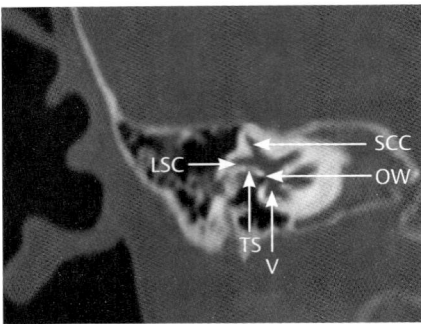

Fig. 4.11 Coronal high-resolution computed tomography (HRCT) of temporal bone showing superior semicircular canal (SCC), lateral semicircular canal (LSC), oval window (OW), tympanic segment of facial nerve (TS), and vestibule (V).

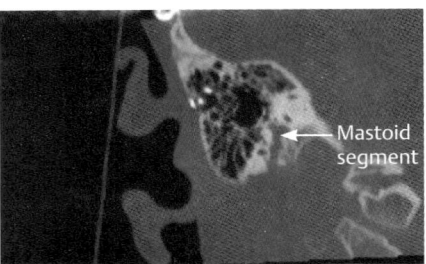

Fig. 4.12 Coronal high-resolution computed tomography (HRCT) of temporal bone showing vertical segment of facial nerve in mastoid part of temporal bone.

Magnetic Resonance Imaging

Fig. 4.13, Fig. 4.14, and **Fig. 4.15** show axial magnetic resonance imaging of brain.

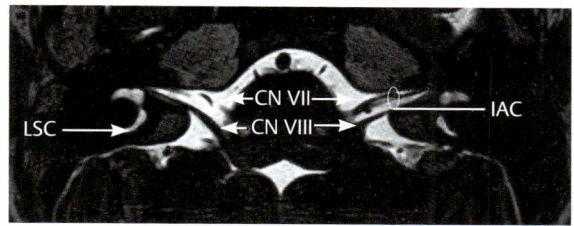

Fig. 4.13 Magnetic resonance imaging (MRI) of brain (T2W) axial section showing cranial nerve VII (facial nerve), cranial nerve VIII (vestibulocochlear nerve), entering internal auditory canal (IAC) from cerebellopontine angle, and lateral semicircular canal (LSC).

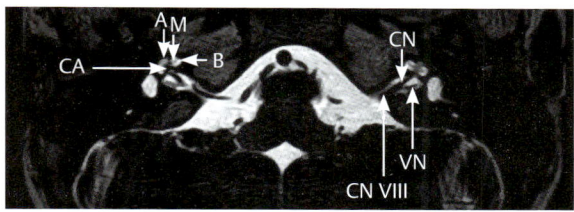

Fig. 4.14 Magnetic resonance imaging (MRI) of brain (T2W) axial section showing cochlea with apical (A), middle (M), and basal (B) turns. CA, cochlear aperture; CN, cochlear nerve; VN, vestibular nerve.

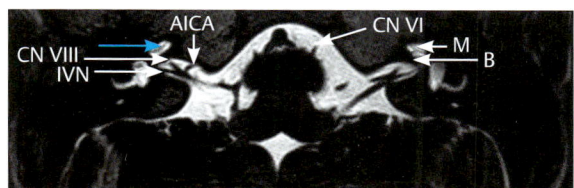

Fig. 4.15 Magnetic resonance imaging (MRI) of brain (T2W) axial section showing cranial nerve VI (facial nerve), cranial nerve VIII (vestibulocochlear nerve), inferior vestibular nerve (IVN), anterior inferior cerebellar artery (AICA), and middle (M) and basal (B) turn of cochlea (*blue arrow* showing osseous spiral lamina).

Facial Nerve Abnormality

Incomplete Partition Deformities

- IP-I and IP-II: Facial nerve has a normal course.
- IP-III and cochlear hypoplasia: Facial nerve has an anomalous course (**Fig. 4.16, Fig. 4.17, Fig. 4.18, Fig. 4.19, Fig. 4.20,** and **Fig. 4.21**).
- A normal lateral semicircular canal is important to have for a normal course of facial nerve. In case of any anomaly in lateral semicircular canal, we need to be cautious during the cochlear implant surgery.

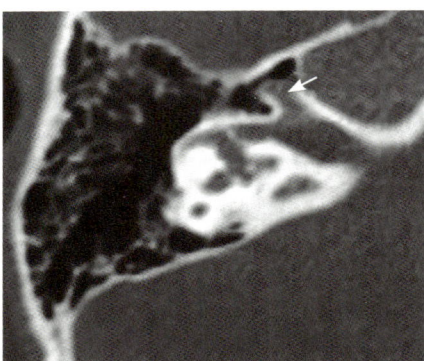

Fig. 4.16 Axial high-resolution computed tomography (HRCT) of temporal bone showing anteriorly displaced labyrinthine segment of facial nerve (*white arrow*).

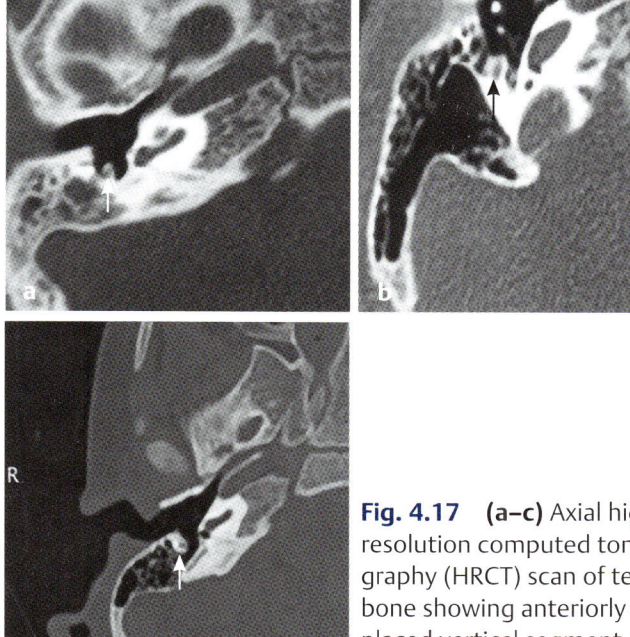

Fig. 4.17 **(a–c)** Axial high-resolution computed tomography (HRCT) scan of temporal bone showing anteriorly displaced vertical segment of facial nerve (*white and black arrow*).

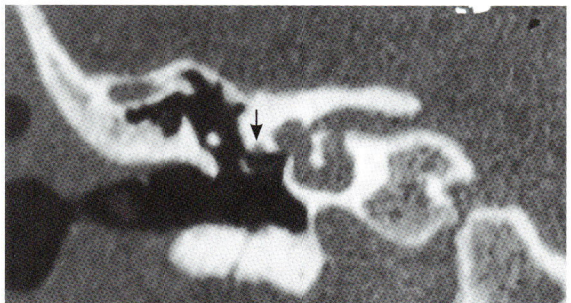

Fig. 4.18 Coronal high-resolution computed tomography (HRCT) of temporal bone showing absent lateral and superior semicircular canals and anteriorly displaced tympanic segment of facial nerve (*black arrow*).

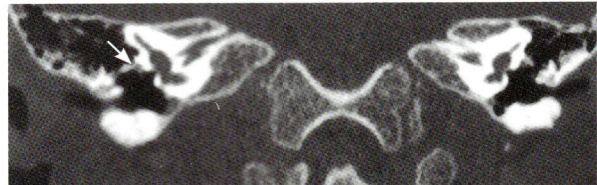

Fig. 4.19 Coronal high-resolution computed tomography (HRCT) of temporal bone showing absent lateral semicircular (LSC) and superiorly displaced tympanic segment of facial nerve (*white arrow*).

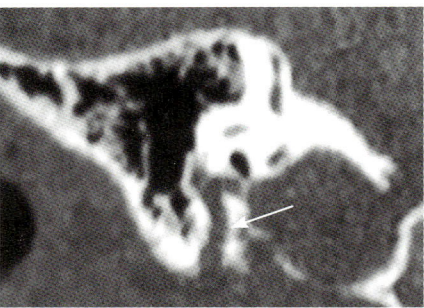

Fig. 4.20 Coronal high-resolution computed tomography (HRCT) of temporal bone showing enlarged facial nerve canal in the mastoid segment (*white arrow*).

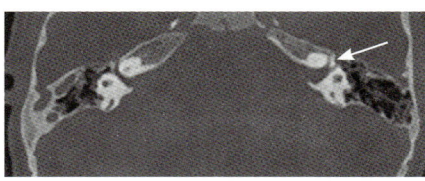

Fig. 4.21 Axial high-resolution computed tomography (HRCT) of temporal bone showing duplication of facial nerve (*white arrow*).

Embryological Development of Facial Nerve

- The complex anatomy of the facial nerve can be best appreciated by studying its embryological development.
- It helps surgeons to understand and anticipate variations.

- The facial nerve develops from otic capsule and second branchial arch (Reichert's cartilage) (all structures developing from second branchial arch are supplied by the facial nerve).
- There is a close relation in development of second arch and otic vesicles, which explains why the developmental changes in the inner ear are associated with facial nerve anomalies.

Case 1

Fig. 4.22, Fig. 4.23, and **Fig. 4.24** show images with absent stapes and facial nerve lying at the oval window.

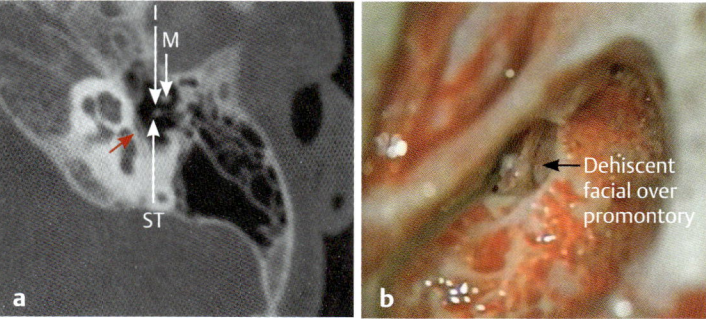

Fig. 4.22 (a, b) Axial high-resolution computed tomography (HRCT) of temporal bone showing left temporal bone, malleus (M), incus (I), and stapedial tendon (ST). Stapes is absent. Facial nerve (*red arrow*) visualized lying over oval window.

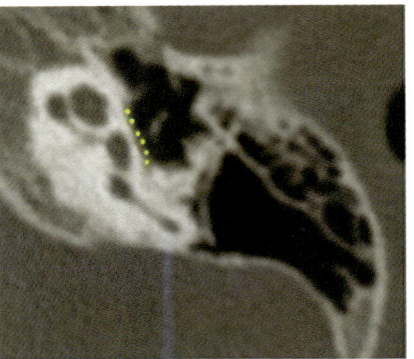

Fig. 4.23 Zoomed image with *yellow dots* showing facial nerve over promontory.

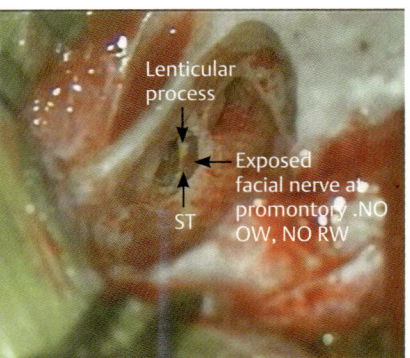

Fig. 4.24 Intraoperative photo of the computed tomography (CT) scan in **Fig. 4.21** where stapedial tendon (ST) is seen attached directly to lenticular process; facial nerve is lying exposed over the promontory. Oval window (OW) and round window (RW).

Facial Nerve in Cochlear Aplasia

Inner ear malformation (cochlear aplasia) has abnormal location of labyrinthine segment of facial nerve due to absence of normal cochlear structures and has aberrant tympanic segment of facial nerve (**Fig. 4.25, Fig. 4.26,** and **Fig. 4.27**).

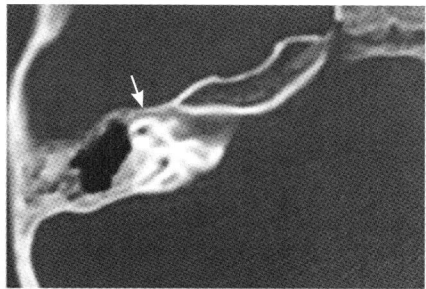

Fig. 4.25 Axial high-resolution computed tomography (HRCT) of temporal bone showing cochlear aplasia with labyrinthine segment of facial nerve anteriorly placed (*white arrow*).

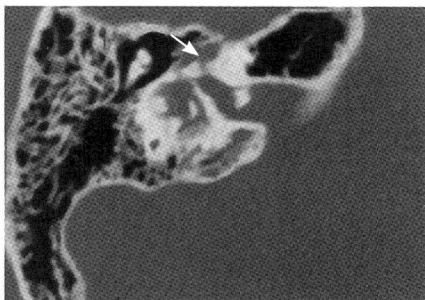

Fig. 4.26 Axial high-resolution computed tomography (HRCT) of temporal bone showing cochlear aplasia with abnormally placed facial nerve (*white arrow*).

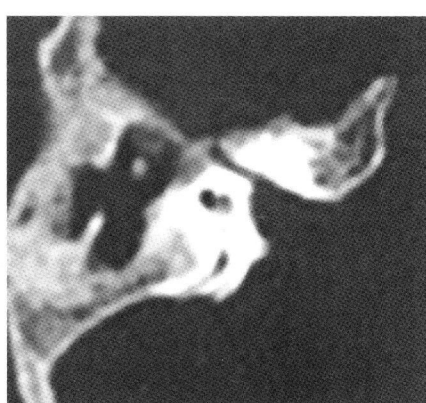

Fig. 4.27 Axial high-resolution computed tomography (HRCT) of temporal bone showing cochlear aplasia with only facial nerve coming out from internal auditory canal (IAC).

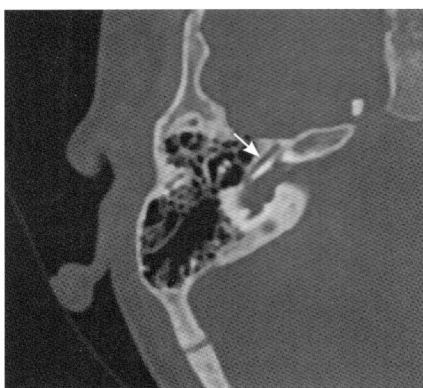

Fig. 4.28 Axial high-resolution computed tomography (HRCT) of temporal bone showing facial nerve (*white arrow*) in common cavity.

Facial Nerve with Common Cavity

Refer **Fig. 4.28**.

Dehiscent Tympanic Segment of Facial Nerve

Refer **Fig. 4.29**.

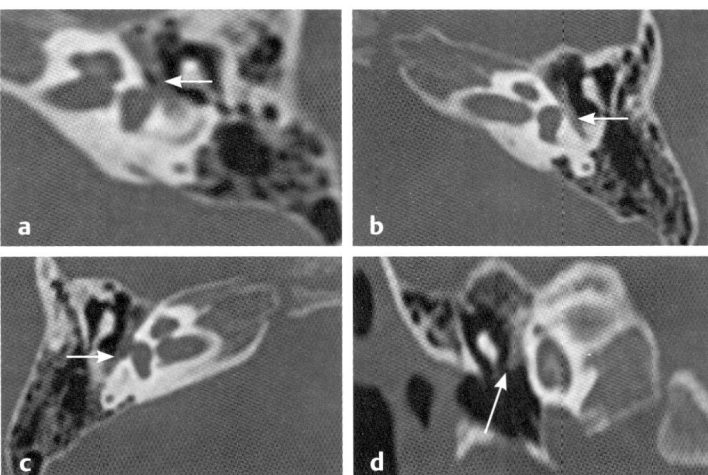

Fig. 4.29 **(a)** Axial high-resolution computed tomography (HRCT) of temporal bone showing dehiscent tympanic segment of facial nerve (*white arrow*). **(b)** Dehiscent facial nerve seen in tympanic segment (*white arrow*). **(c)** Dehiscent facial nerve tympanic part (*white arrow*). **(d)** Coronal HRCT of temporal bone showing dehiscent facial nerve seen in tympanic segment (*white arrow*).

Facial Nerve Injury

- Heat injury can occur during extensive drilling especially in ossification cases, which can lead to neural edema, further leading to vasodilatation. Narrow space between posterior tympanotomy and round window brings the burr closer to the nerve and increases the risk of heat dissipation (**Fig. 4.30** and **Fig. 4.31**).

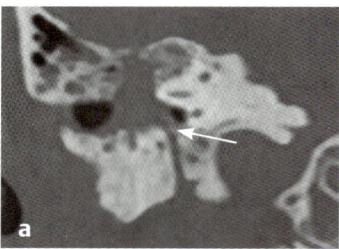 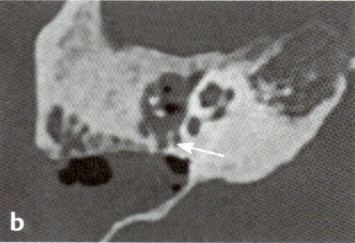

Fig. 4.30 **(a)** High-resolution computed tomography (HRCT) of temporal bone coronal section showing injury at facial canal (*white arrow*) in a case of cochlear implant at the second genu. **(b)** Axial HRCT of temporal bone showing injury at mastoid segment of facial nerve (*white arrow*).

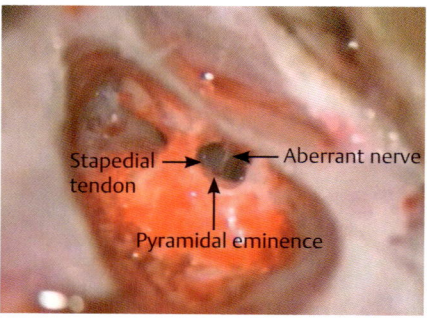

Fig. 4.31 Intraoperative photograph showing stapedial tendon, pyramidal eminence, and an aberrant nerve originating from pyramidal eminence.

- Reasons for late-onset facial nerve palsy are:
  - Acute nerve compromise (from vasospasm).
  - Reactivation of herpes virus resulting from surgical trauma.
  - Manipulation and transection of chorda tympani nerve.

Precautions

The primary goal is to avoid complications.

- Know the anatomy.
- Read the imaging.
- Use facial nerve monitor (it can help limit potential nerve damage).
- Apply copious irrigation.
- While drilling the round window niche burr should be angled. So the drill shaft is held away from the facial nerve.

Case 2
Duplication of Facial Nerve

Facial nerve runs inside the bony canal, hence making the canal visible on computed tomography (CT) (**Fig. 4.32** and **Fig. 4.33**).

- The facial nerve has been marked by yellow dots showing the duplication of vertical segment of the facial nerve during its course.

Coronal Section

- The facial nerve has been marked by yellow dots showing the duplication of vertical segment of the facial nerve during its course.

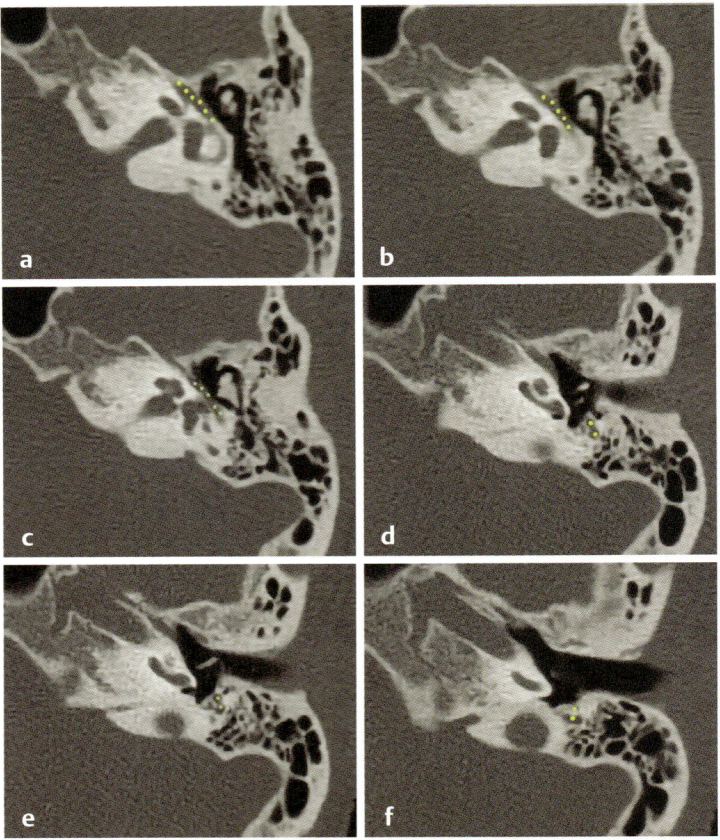

Fig. 4.32 High-resolution computed tomography (HRCT) of temporal bone (axial scan) showing **(a)** labyrinthine segment seen with the first genu. **(b, c)** Tympanic segment. **(d–f)** Duplication of mastoid part of facial nerve. *Yellow dots* signifies the tract of facial nerve from up to down in the scan which is then showing duplication in the mastoid segment.

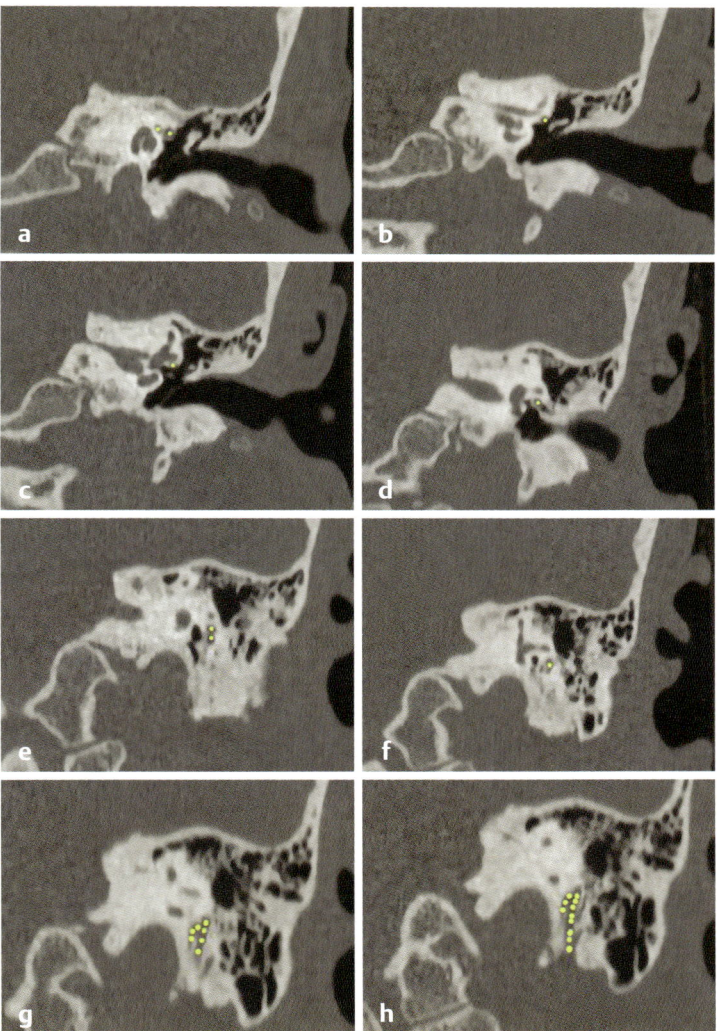

Fig. 4.33 High-resolution computed tomography (HRCT) of temporal bone (coronal scans). **(a)** Labyrinthine and tympanic segments are seen as two dots. **(b–d)** Tympanic segment. **(e–h)** Duplication of vertical segment.

59

Case 3

Fig. 4.34 shows HRCT of temporal bone axial sections with displaced facial nerve lying directly over the promontory (series of scan, superior to inferior).

- The facial nerve has been marked by yellow dots showing displaced facial nerve lying over the promontory during its course.

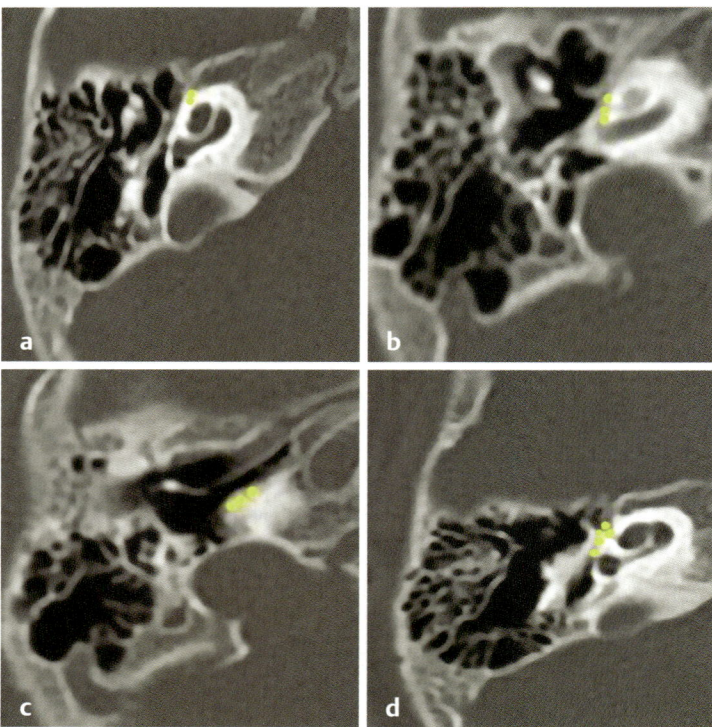

Fig. 4.34 (a–d) High-resolution computed tomography (HRCT) of temporal bone (axial scans) showing abnormal placement of the facial nerve over the promontory. *Yellow dots* signifies the tract of facial nerve from up to down in the scan showing abnormal placement.

Management

- If injury is noted intraoperatively (severe enough to warrant repair), repair with primary reanastomosis or cable graft.
- If injury is noted in immediate postoperative period with high suspicion of direct injury, proceed for repair (especially grade 4). If the surgeon knows the nerve was intact, treat it with steroids and antiviral medications.
- Late onset of facial paresis:
  - Treatment with steroids: Start with 60 mg prednisolone for 10 days and then taper for a total of 21 days.

We had late-onset facial paresis in three cases in adult cochlear implantation (all were females).

- Last but not the least, in facial nerve and cochlear implants, facial nerve stimulation can occur following implantation.
  - Due to current spread within the electrode (can lead to spread of current from the electrode to the facial nerve).
  - The pathways of spread of current are:
    - ○ Cochlear nerve via scala tympani.
    - ○ Spread along bony canal to adjacent structure (labyrinthine segment crosses the basal turn of cochlea close to the scala tympani so it is close to electrode array).

Conclusion

- There is increased incidence of stimulation in oto-sclerosis due to spongiotic bone leading to decreased impedance to current spread within the normal bone.
- Facial nerve paresis and stimulation are potential complications in cochlear implant surgery.
- Knowledge of facial nerve anomalies is of utmost importance.
- Avoid exposing facial nerve in facial recess area.

Suggested Reading

Sennaroğlu L. Cochlear implantation in inner ear malformations—a review article. Cochlear Implants Int 2010;11(1):4–41

Sennaroğlu L, Özkan HB, Aslan F. Impact of cochleovestibular malformations in treating children with hearing loss. Cochlear (TM) Science and Research Seminar; 2013; İstanbul, Turkey, pp. 23–27

Sennaroğlu L, Tahir E. A Novel Classification: Anomalous Routes of the Facial Nerve in Relation to Inner Ear Malformations. Laryngoscope. 2020 Nov;130(11):E696-E703

Sennaroğlu L, Ziyal I, Atas A, et al. Preliminary results of auditory brainstem implantation in prelingually deaf children with inner ear malformations including severe stenosis of the cochlear aperture and aplasia of the cochlear nerve. Otol Neurotol 2009;30(6):708–715

5 Cochlear Abnormalities

Introduction

It is estimated that 20% of all children with congenital sensory neural hearing loss present with inner ear malformations (IEMs). Inner ear anomalies still pose a significant challenge for the surgeon, audiologist, and speech language pathologist. Currently many centers prefer not to implant IEM patients due to uncertainty in auditory outcomes and increased risk of surgical complications (perilymph leak, cerebrospinal fluid (CSF) gusher, injuring facial nerve, and electrode array migration). Due to anomalous and reduced neural tissue distribution in IEM, the outcomes cannot be predicted.

Embryology of Cochlea

In order to understand cochlear anomaly, we need to understand the development of cochlea in the embryonic stage (**Fig. 5.1, Fig. 5.2,** and **Fig. 5.3**).

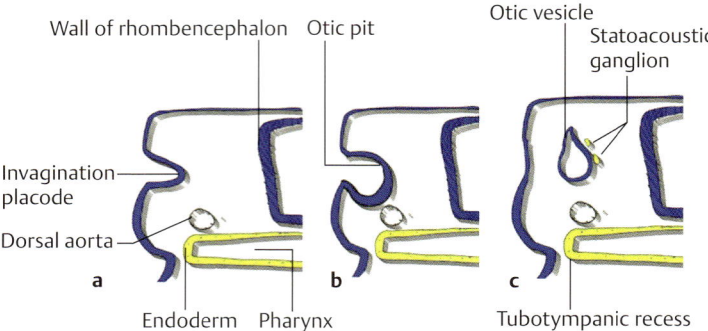

Fig. 5.1 **(a)** Surface ectoderm forms a short-lived thickening, the otic placode, dorsolateral to the hind brain. **(b)** Otic placode invaginates into mesenchyme adjacent to rhombencephalon to form otic pit. **(c)** The folds of otic pit fuse together to form otic vesicle, enveloped by mesenchyme to form otic capsule. Stratoacoustic ganglion arises as neurons delaminate and later the ganglion splits into cochlear and vestibular portions.

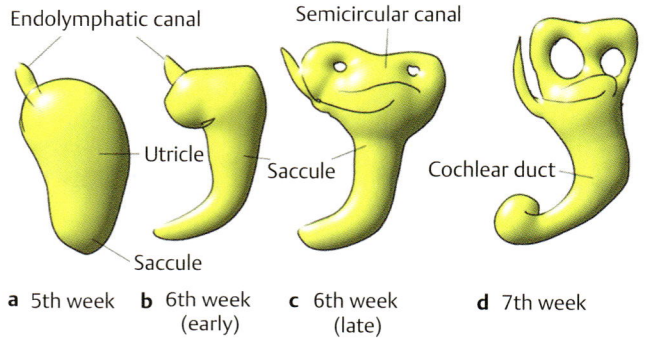

Fig. 5.2 **(a)** Otic vesicle forms two visible regions: ventral saccular portion and dorsal utricular portion. **(b)** Ventral saccular portion give rise to cochlea and saccule, dorsal utricular portion give rise to utricle and semicircular canals. **(c)** They further differentiate into anterior and posterior saccule. **(d)** Ventral portion further forms the cochlear duct.

64

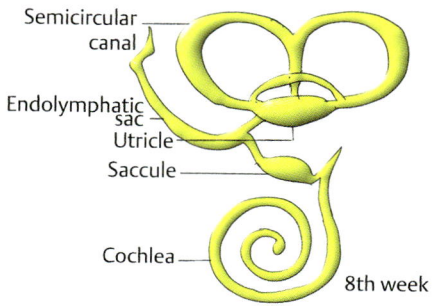

Fig. 5.3 Well-formed and differentiated inner ear has utricle, anterior, posterior, and lateral semicircular canal attached to it. Endolymphatic sac is connected to saccule and cochlear duct.

Cochlear Anomaly

Cochlear malformations are a challenge to the surgeon. Knowing the imaging well helps in differentiating normal from abnormal. It guides and prepares the surgeon intraoperatively about complications that can happen and how to prevent and prepare in the operating room (OR) (**Flowchart 5.1**).

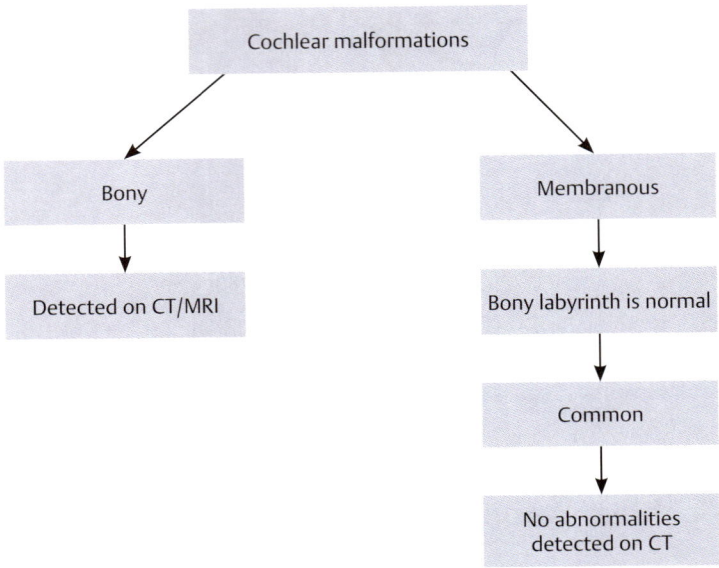

Flowchart 5.1 Types of cochlear malformations.

Classification of Anomaly

An imaging-based classification was first proposed in 1987 by Jackler et al.[1] However, Sennaroglu et al[2] later refined the classification and its pathophysiological basis using computed tomography (CT). The latest classification by Sennaroglu (2017) is the most commonly used.

The two classifications of cochlear anomaly are described in **Table 5.1**.

Table 5.1 Classification of cochlear anomaly

Jackler (1987)	Sennaroglu (2017)
Michel deformity	Complete labyrinthine aplasia (Michel deformity): • With hypoplastic or aplastic petrous bone • Without otic capsule • With otic capsule
Cochlear aplasia	Rudimentary otocyst
Common cavity	Cochlear aplasia: • With normal (vestibular) labyrinth • With dilated vestibule • Common cavity
Incomplete partition (mild)/Mondini deformity	Cochlear hypoplasia (types I–IV): • Bud-like cochlea (CH-I) • Cystic hypoplastic cochlea (CH-II) • Cochlea with less than two turns (CH-III) • Cochlea with hypoplastic middle and apical turns (CH-IV)
Cochlear hypoplasia (mild)	Incomplete partition type I (IP-I; cystic cochleovestibular anomaly)
Incomplete partition (severe)	Incomplete partition type II (IP-II, including as part of the Mondini malformation)
Cochlear hypoplasia (severe)	Incomplete partition type III (IP-III; X-linked deafness)
	Enlarged vestibular aqueduct
	Cochlear aperture abnormalities: • Hypoplasia • Aplasia

Michel Deformity/Complete Labyrinthine Aplasia

Michel aplasia is thought to result from failure of development of the otic placode, due to developmental arrest at the third week of gestation. It is the most severe kind of malformation. It is therefore a contraindication for cochlear implantation (**Fig. 5.4**).

Rudimentary Otocyst

Rudimentary otocyst, as the name suggests, results due to failure of development of inner ear after otocyst stage. Single small cavity is visualized in petrous bone which may not connect to the internal auditory canal (IAC) (**Fig. 5.5**).

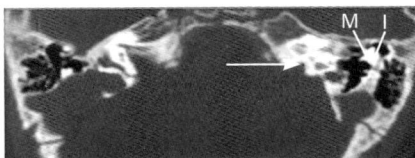

Fig. 5.4 Computed tomography (CT) of temporal bone axial cut showing incus (I) and malleus (M) bones but complete absence of cochlea and semicircular canals (*white arrow*).

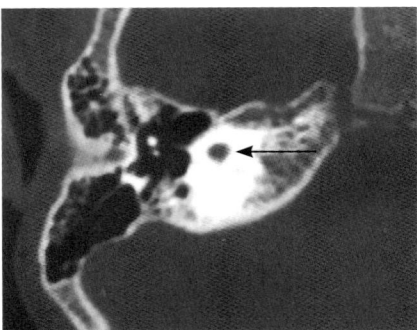

Fig. 5.5 High-resolution computed tomography (HRCT) axial scan showing incomplete representation of otic capsule without internal auditory canal (IAC) (*black arrow*).

Cochlear Aplasia

- In this case the cochlea is absent, but the vestibule is developed with either cochlear aplasia with vestibular dilatation (CAVD) or well-formed semicircular canals (3rd to 4th weeks of gestation) (**Fig. 5.6** and **Fig. 5.7**).
- For identification purpose we use the dictum: **Anything below IAC is vestibule and above IAC is cochlea**.
- Cochlear aplasia is a contraindication to cochlear implant.

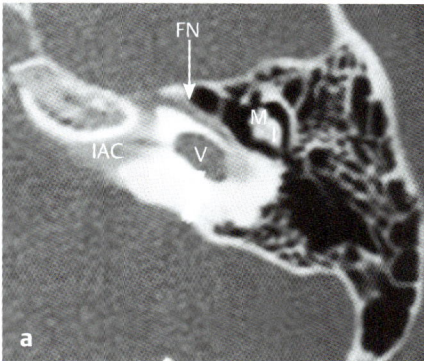
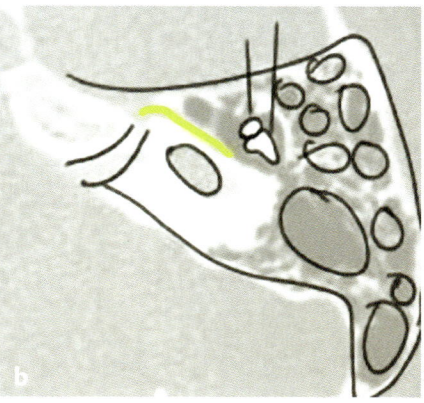

Fig. 5.6 **(a)** High-resolution computed tomography (HRCT) axial image showing the internal auditory canal (IAC), facial nerve (FN), dilated vestibule (V) below IAC, and ear ossicles incus (I) and malleus (M). **(b)** A schematic diagram of the same HRCT image showing facial nerve (*yellow line*) and ear ossicles (*black arrows*).

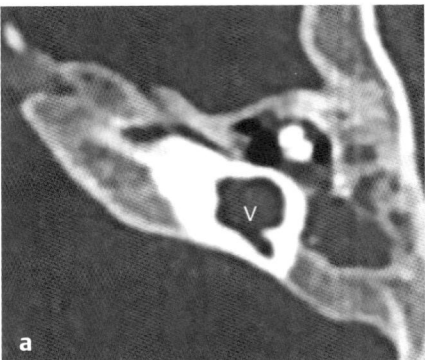

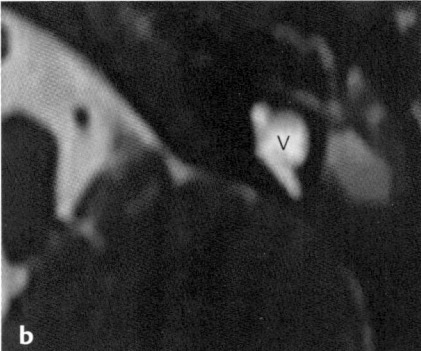

Fig. 5.7 **(a)** Axial high-resolution computed tomography (HRCT) showing dilated dysplastic vestibule (V) with ear ossicles. **(b)** T2 magnetic resonance imaging (MRI) of the same cut showing fluid-filled vestibule.

Common Cavity

A common cavity malformation is due to an arrest in development in the 4th week of gestation. In a common cavity there is one single cavity, representing cochlea and vestibule, without any differentiation into cochlear and vestibular structures. If the cavity is located at the posterior side of the IAC, then there is no distinction between common cavity and a cochlear aplasia (**Fig. 5.8, Fig. 5.9, Fig. 5.10,** and **Fig. 5.11**).

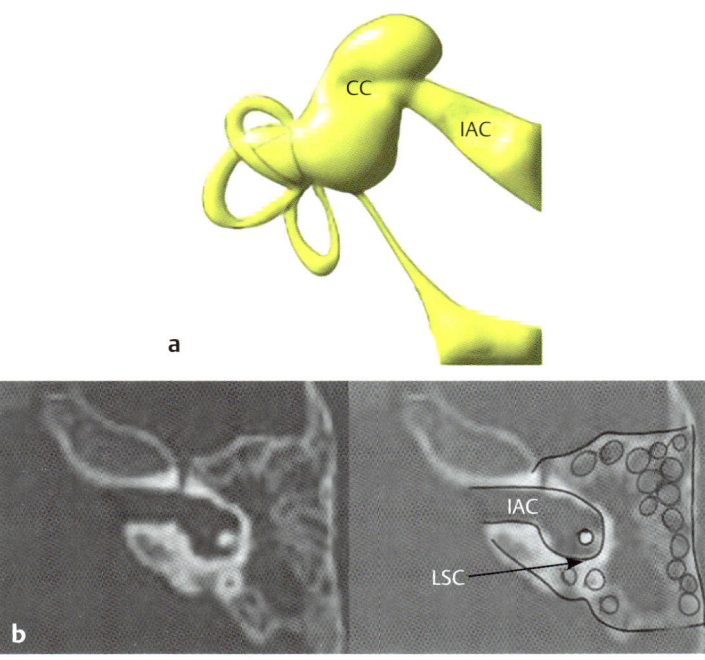

Fig. 5.8 **(a)** Schematic diagram of inner ear showing the internal auditory canal (IAC) is directly connected to the common cystic cavity (CC). **(b)** Image showing IAC is directly connected to the cystic cavity and lateral semicircular canal.

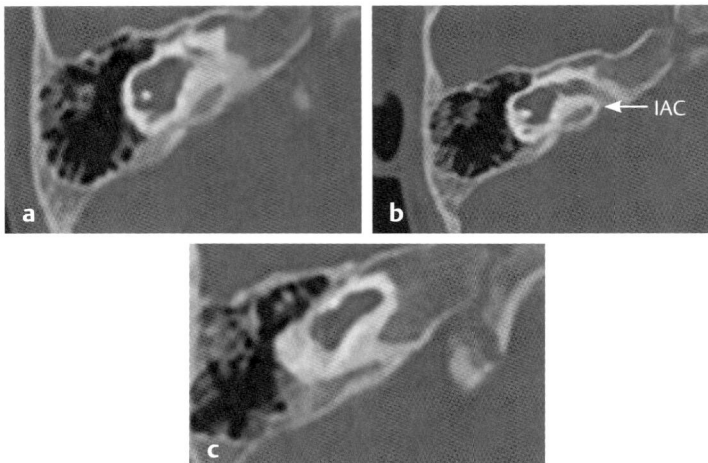

Fig. 5.9 High-resolution computed tomography (HRCT) axial scan of common cavity. **(a)** Section above the level of the internal auditory canal (IAC) looks like dilated vestibule with lateral semicircular canal (SCC). **(b)** At the level of the IAC it looks like the cavity is continuous with the IAC. **(c)** Below the level of the IAC it looks like a large cavity without any bony septa.

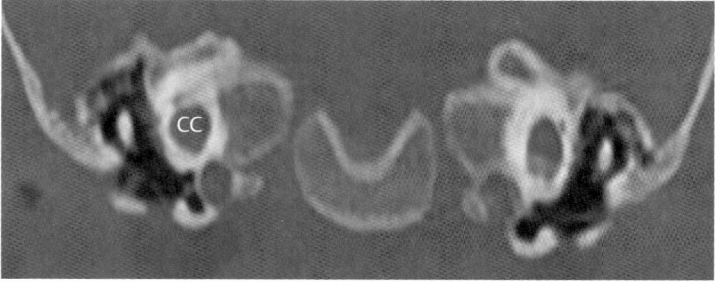

Fig. 5.10 High-resolution computed tomography (HRCT) coronal scan of common cavity (CC) showing a single cavity in the petrous region.

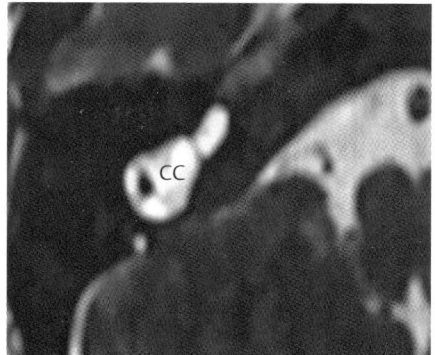

Fig. 5.11 Magnetic resonance imaging (MRI) T2 sequence of common cavity (CC).

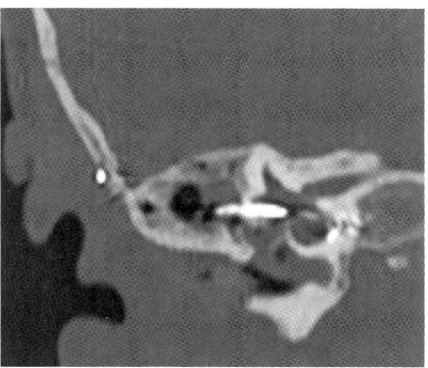

Fig. 5.12 High-resolution computed tomography (HRCT) coronal section showing implant entering through lateral semicircular canal.

Common Cavity Post Cochlear Implant

- Cochlear implantation in common cavity is through translabyrinthine route.
- As whole cochlea and vestibule comprises a single cavity, implant is inserted via lateral semicircular canal (**Fig. 5.12** and **Fig. 5.13**).

73

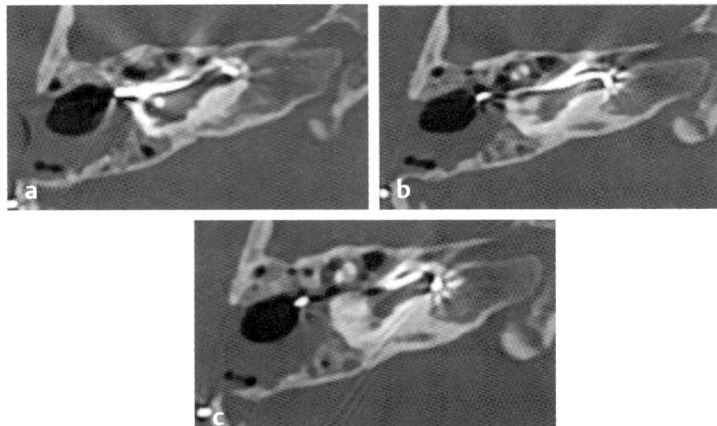

Fig. 5.13 High-resolution computed tomography (HRCT) axial image showing **(a)** implant array entering the cavity via lateral semicircular canal (LSC), **(b)** implant array making a curve in cavity (there is risk of array entering to the internal auditory canal [IAC] in common cavity), and **(c)** array sitting inside the cavity.

Incomplete Partition I (IP-I)

In this type of malformation, the cochlear development arrest occurs in the 5th week of development resulting in a cystic cochlea and vestibule. The modiolus is completely absent and the cochlea does not have interscalar septi. There is a 50% chance of CSF gusher (**Fig. 5.14, Fig. 5.15,** and **Fig. 5.16**).

Fig. 5.17, Fig. 5.18, Fig. 5.19, and **Fig. 5.20** show series of axial CT scan of IP-I from above to downwards.

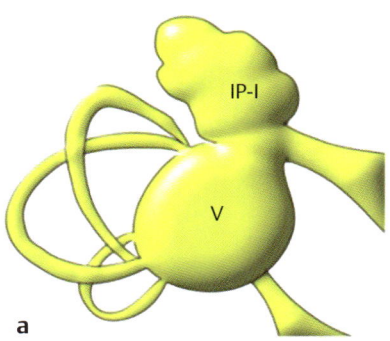

a

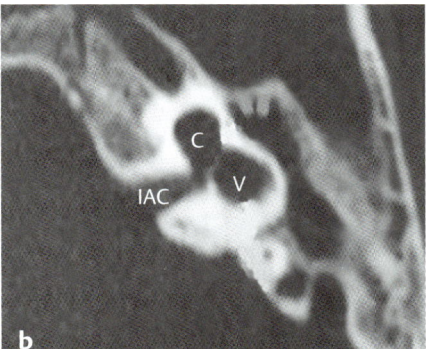

b

Fig. 5.14 **(a)** Clip art diagram of incomplete partition I (IP-I) showing dilated vestibule (V), dilated cochlea with absent modiolus and septi. **(b)** Axial scan of IP-I showing figure-of-8 appearance due to dilated cochlea (C) as well as vestibule with prominent separation in between them. Internal auditory canal (IAC).

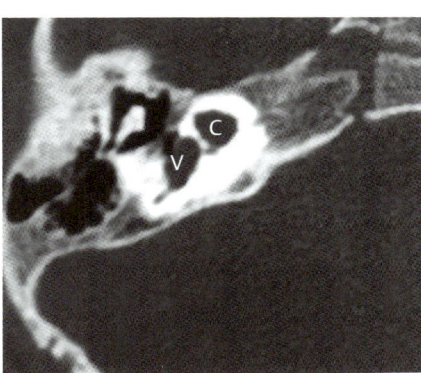

Fig. 5.15 High-resolution computed tomography (HRCT) axial scan of temporal bone with ear ossicles. In this cut there are two cystic swellings, cochlea above (C) and vestibule below (V). Cochlea is without modiolus.

75

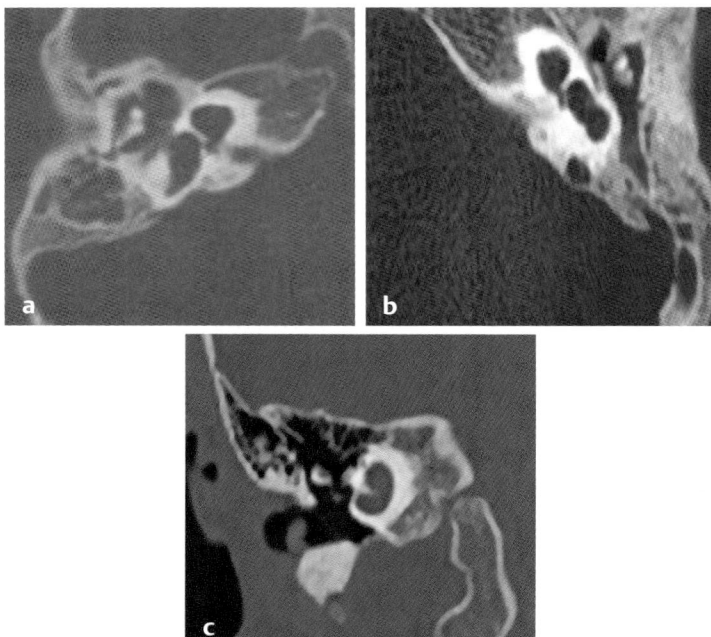

Fig. 5.16 **(a, b)** Axial high-resolution computed tomography (HRCT) of temporal bone showing incomplete partition I (IP-I) deformity. **(c)** HRCT coronal section showing IP-I deformity.

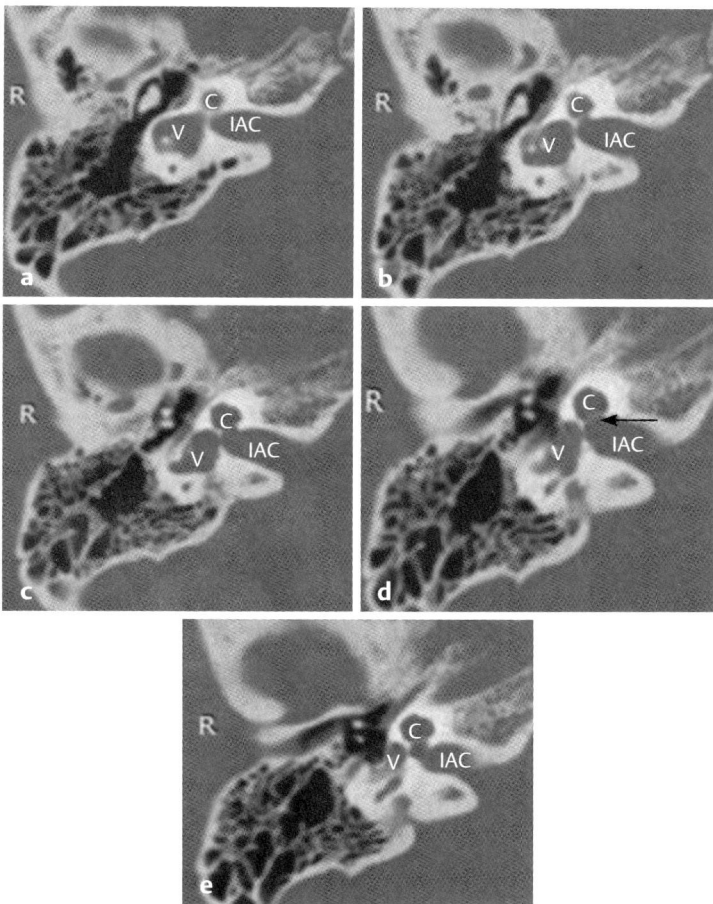

Fig. 5.17 High-resolution computed tomography (HRCT) scan axial section from above downwards showing **(a)** dilated vestibule (V), **(b)** appearance of cochlea (C) (note the lack of modiolus), and **(c)** dilated internal auditory canal (IAC), cochlea, and vestibule. Facial nerve is also seen (tympanic segment). **(d)** Cystic cochlea with IAC and cribriform (*black arrow*) between them visible (unlike common cavity). **(e)** Crura of stapes visible with incus and malleus, dilated cystic cochlea.

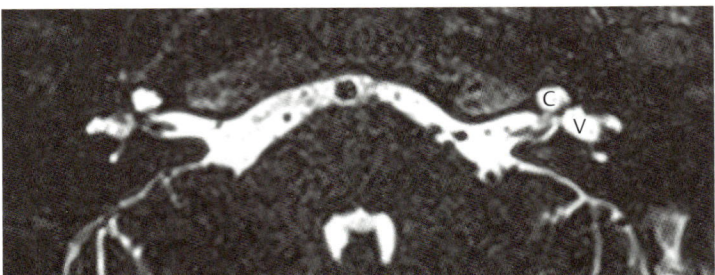

Fig. 5.18 Magnetic resonance imaging (MRI) T2 sequence of temporal bone axial scan showing incomplete partition I (IP-I) cystic cochlea (C) without modiolus and dilated vestibule (V).

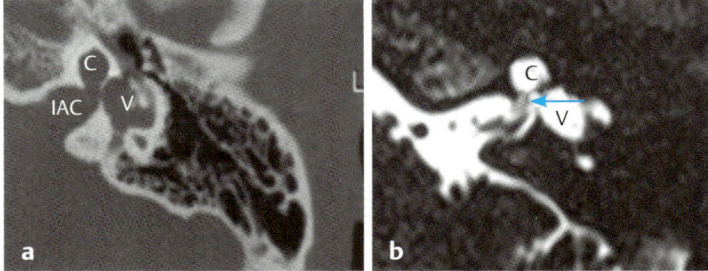

Fig. 5.19 **(a)** High-resolution computed tomography (HRCT) of temporal bone axial image showing the internal auditory canal (IAC) and cystic cochlea (C) with dilated vestibule (V). **(b)** Magnetic resonance imaging (MRI) T2 sequence showing the same cut with cochlear nerve (*blue arrow*) going inside cochlea.

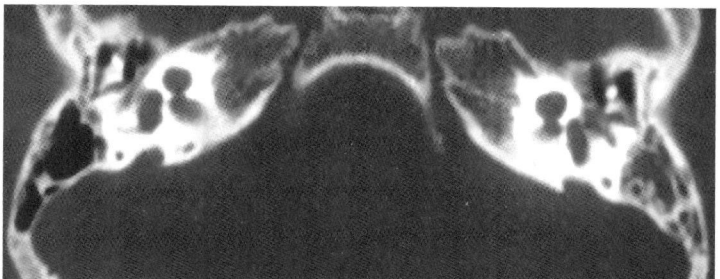

Fig. 5.20 High-resolution computed tomography (HRCT) of temporal bone axial section showing cochlear hypoplasia-II on right side and incomplete partition I on left side.

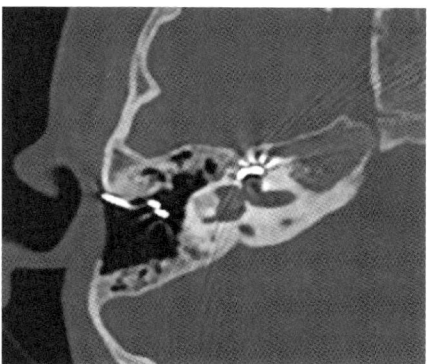

Fig. 5.21 Axial high-resolution computed tomography (HRCT) scan of post cochlear implantation ear showing electrode array in cochlea.

IP-I Post Cochlear Implant

Fig. 5.21 and **Fig. 5.22** shows array placed well in the IP-I case with no curling or misplacement.

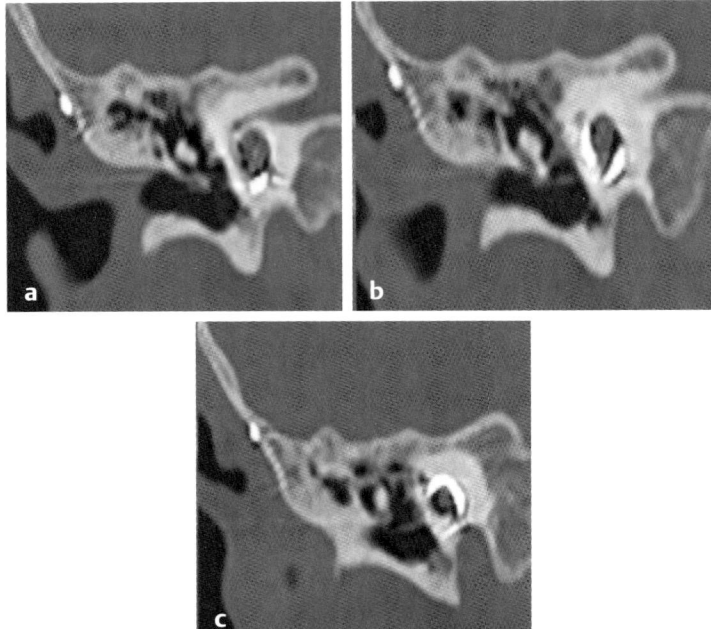

Fig. 5.22 (a–c) Coronal high-resolution computed tomography (HRCT) scan showing electrode array in cochlea.

Mondini (IP-II)

Refer **Fig. 5.23, Fig. 5.24, Fig. 5.25, Fig. 5.26, Fig. 5.27, Fig. 5.28, Fig. 5.29, Fig. 5.30, Fig. 5.31, Fig. 5.32, Fig. 5.33, Fig. 5.34,** and **Fig. 5.35**.

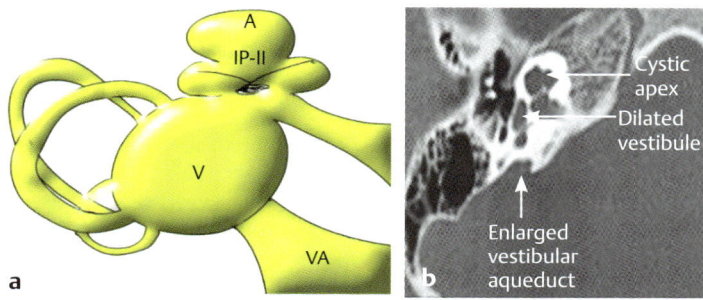

Fig. 5.23 **(a)** Clip art diagram of incomplete partition II (IP-II) showing cystic apex (A) of cochlea enlarged vestibule (V), and enlarged vestibular aqueduct (VA). **(b)** High-resolution computed tomography (HRCT) of temporal bone axial section showing cystic middle and apical turn of cochlea, dilated vestibule, and enlarged vestibular aqueduct (Mondini triad). Please note all the structures do not appear in the same cut in axial scan; we need to look them at different levels.

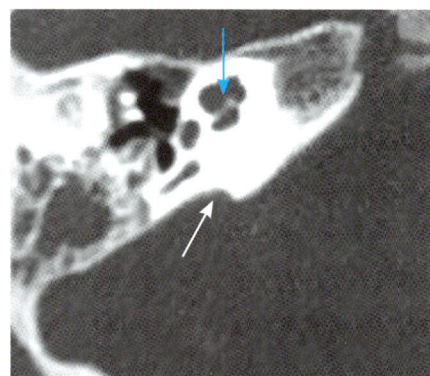

Fig. 5.24 High-resolution computed tomography (HRCT) of temporal bone axial section showing cystic apical and middle turns of cochlea (*blue arrow*) and vestibular aqueduct (*white arrow*).

81

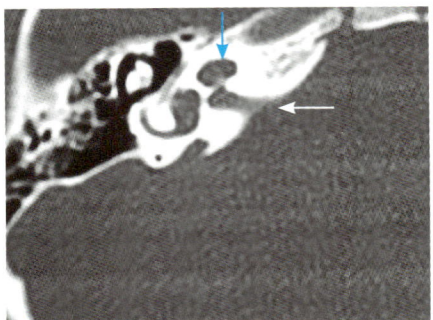

Fig. 5.25 High-resolution computed tomography (HRCT) of temporal bone axial cut showing cystic cochlear apex (*blue arrow*) triad with narrow internal auditory canal (IAC) (*white arrow*).

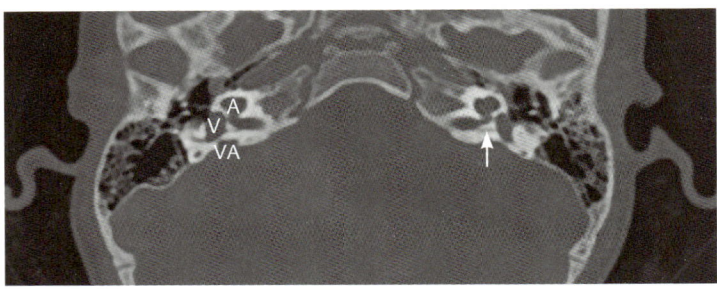

Fig. 5.26 Image showing cystic apex (A), dilated vestibule (V), enlarged vestibular aqueduct (VA), and singular nerve (*white arrow*).

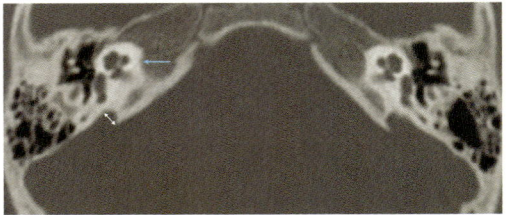

Fig. 5.27 High-resolution computed tomography (HRCT) of temporal bone axial section showing cystic apical and middle turn with normal basal turn (*blue arrow*), and enlarged vestibular aqueduct (*white arrow*).

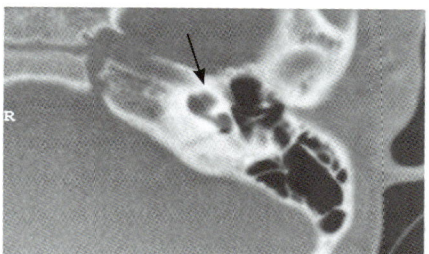

Fig. 5.28 High-resolution computed tomography (HRCT) of temporal bone showing a cystic apex (*black arrow*).

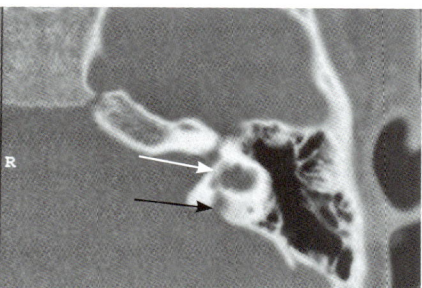

Fig. 5.29 Axial section showing dilated vestibule and large vestibular aqueduct (*white and black arrows*).

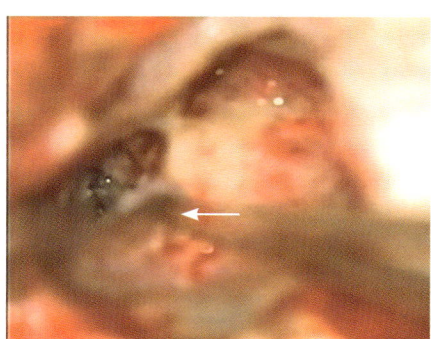

Fig. 5.30 Fascia is harvested, and electrode array is passed through the fascia for sealing the cerebrospinal fluid (CSF) leak at the round window.

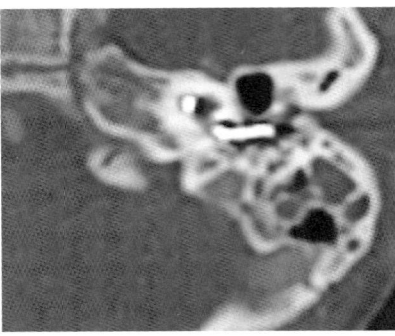

Fig. 5.31 High-resolution computed tomography (HRCT) of temporal bone axial section showing postoperative cochlear implant electrode in a patient with Mondini dysplasia with cerebrospinal fluid (CSF) in the middle ear and mastoid cavity.

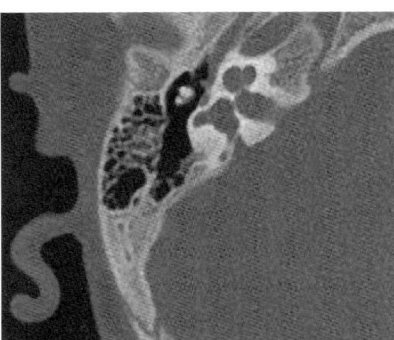

Fig. 5.32 High-resolution computed tomography (HRCT) axial section of a case of incomplete partition II (IP-II) with microtia.

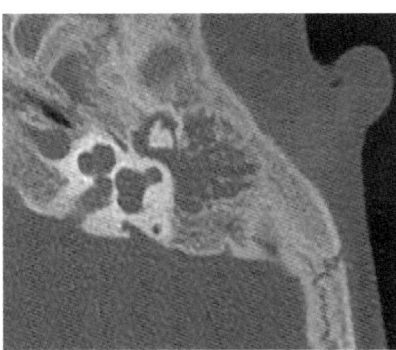

Fig. 5.33 High-resolution computed tomography (HRCT) of temporal bone axial scan showing lack of external ear and external auditory canal (EAC) (anotia), with Mondini triad.

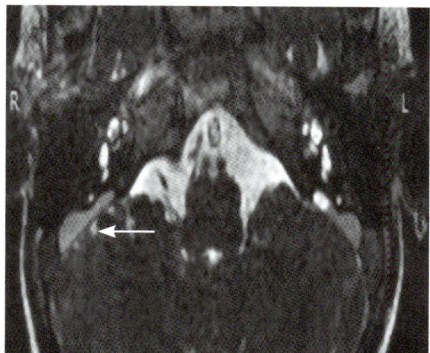

Fig. 5.34 Magnetic resonance imaging (MRI) axial section showing endolymphatic sac (*white arrow*).

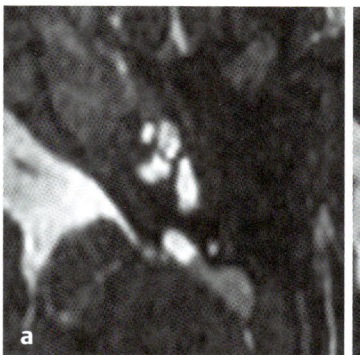

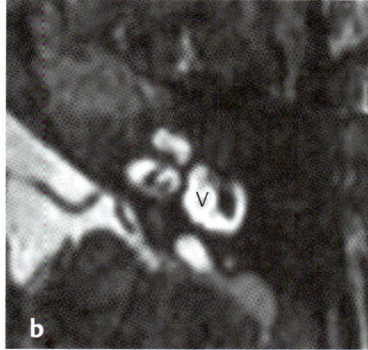

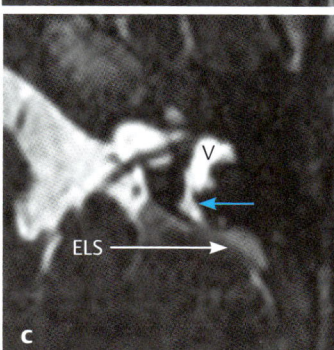

Fig. 5.35 Magnetic resonance imaging (MRI) T2 sequence. **(a)** Cystic apical and middle turn with vestibular space dilated. **(b)** Basal turn of cochlea and dilated vestibule (V), with enlarged aqueduct. **(c)** Vestibular aqueduct connected to vestibule (*blue arrow*), internal auditory canal (IAC) with nerve. ELS, endolymphatic sac (*white arrow*).

Incomplete Partition III (IP-III)

IP-III is usually X-linked disorder; the septa are present but modiolus is absent (**Fig. 5.36, Fig. 5.37,** and **Fig. 5.38**).

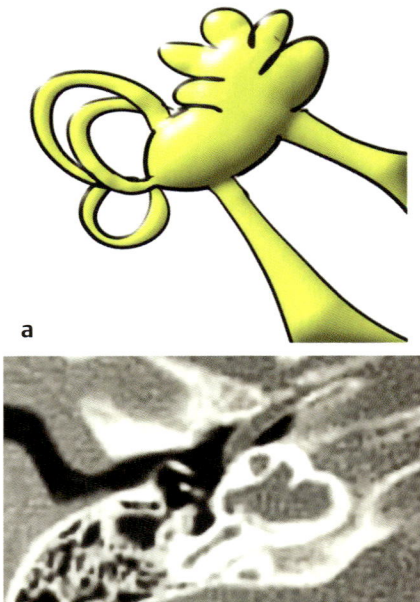

Fig. 5.36 **(a)** Clip art of incomplete partition III (IP-III) showing presence of septa but lack of modiolus. **(b)** High-resolution computed tomography (HRCT) of temporal bone axial section showing the same findings in **(a)**.

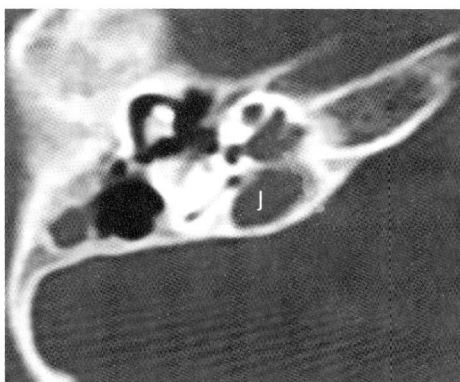

Fig. 5.37 High-resolution computed tomography (HRCT) of temporal bone axial image showing interscalar septa in cochlea without modiolus and high jugular bulb (J).

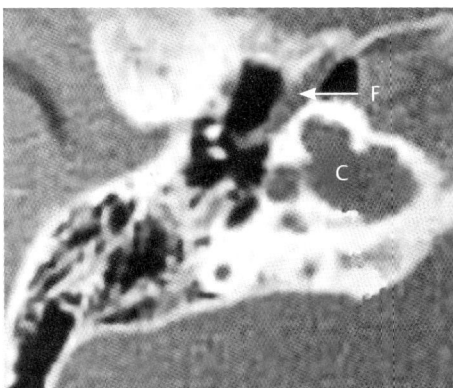

Fig. 5.38 High-resolution computed tomography (HRCT) of temporal bone axial section showing Christmas tree appearance of cochlea (C) with tympanic segment of facial nerve (F).

Comparison of Cochlear Anomalies (Fig. 5.39)

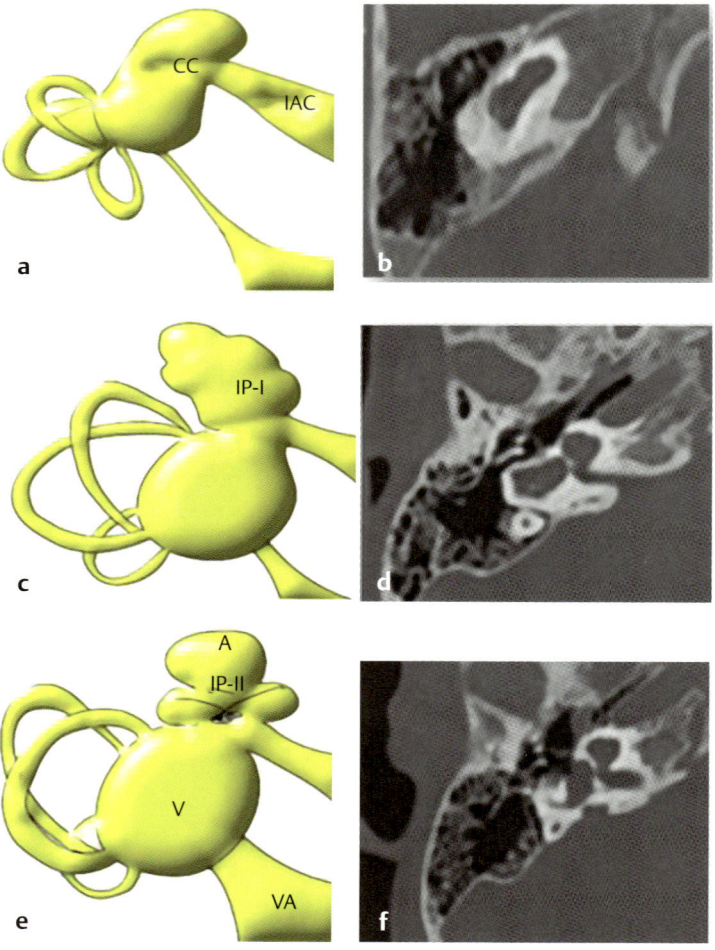

Fig. 5.39 (a–f) Comparison of various cochlear anomalies. Abbreviations: CC, Common cavity; IAC, internal auditory canal; V, vestibule; VA, vestibular aqueduct. *(continued)*

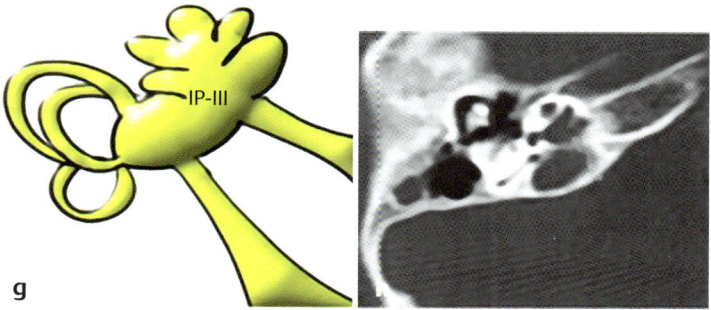

g

Fig. 5.39 *(continued)* **(g-h)** Comparison of various cochlear anomalies.

References

1. Jackler RK, Luxford WM, House WF. Congenital malformations of the inner ear: a classification based on embryogenesis. Laryngoscope. 1987 Mar;97(3 Pt 2 Suppl 40):2-14
2. Sennaroğlu L, Bajin MD. Classification and Current Management of Inner Ear Malformations. Balkan Med J. 2017 Sep 29;34(5):397-411

5a Cochlear Implant in IP-III Malformation

Introduction

Inner ear anomalies have always posed a serious challenge to radiologists, otologists, and rehabilitation teams alike. For a long time, cochlear implant (CI) surgeries were avoided in IEMs due to multiple intraoperative risks, coupled with uncertain audiological outcomes. First described by Nance et al (1971), incomplete partition type III (IP-III) is one of the rarest malformations with overall incidence of 2%. Inheritance pattern of IP-III is X linked and it presents with profound symmetrical mixed hearing loss.[1] It is associated with mutations in the POU3F4 gene.[2] Stapes footplate fixation leads to conductive hearing loss but is often masked by the sensorineural component. This deformity was included under the category of incomplete partition (IP) by Sennaroglu et al in their landmark publication in 2006.[3] They established that the interscalar septa are present, but the modiolus is completely absent.

The features of IP-III on high-resolution computed tomography (HRCT) of the temporal bone are:

- Christmas tree appearance of the cochlea.
- Dilated IAC.
- Deficient modiolus with lack of partitioning bone (lamina cribrosa) between the IAC and basal turn of the cochlea resulting in wide communication between perilymph of the cochlea and the subarachnoid space (IAC) (**Fig. 5.40**). This leads to increased perilymphatic pressure, which explains the severe CSF gusher on opening the cochlea.
- The external dimensions of the cochlea were found to be similar to the cochlea.
- The labyrinthine segment of the facial nerve is located anteriorly instead of making a gentle curve around the basal turn on axial sections (**Fig. 5.41**).

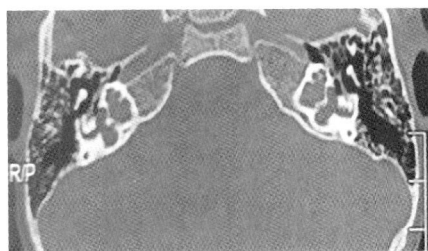

Fig. 5.40 Axial high-resolution computed tomography (HRCT) of temporal bone showing bilateral absence of modiolus.

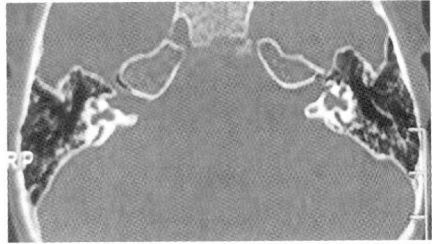

Fig. 5.41 Axial high-resolution computed tomography (HRCT) of temporal bone showing wide internal auditory canal (IAC) with anteriorly placed labyrinthine segment of facial nerve.

There are various perioperative risks associated with cochlear implant surgeries in these patients. Malposition of the electrode array into the IAC is a known complication due to absence of a modiolar base. Patients face an increased risk of postoperative meningitis due to CSF gusher. Sometimes, the surgery becomes more challenging due to the anomalous course of the facial nerve and increased risk of injury to the nerve. With improved surgical strategies and successful auditory rehabilitation in IP-III patients, cochlear implantation is now being considered a standard of care in these candidates.

Clinical Cases—Our Surgical Technique

A total of seven patients underwent primary surgery at our center. One patient was operated at a different center, which was referred to us later. In the first case done at our center, initially intraoperative neural response telemetry (NRT) recording was not found. Intraoperative X-ray (Stenvers view) using a C-arm was done, and it was found that there was a tip fold over inside the cochlea. Hence, it was retrieved and reinserted by slightly bending the electrode array and it was pushed along the lateral wall of the cochlea, taking care not to damage the electrodes. NRT was re-checked and recorded in all electrodes. In all our subsequent cases we followed the same technique of bending the electrode array to align with lateral wall of cochlea in order to avoid malposition into the IAC.

The patient referred to us lacked a recordable NRT with no improvement in audiological outcomes 6 months after the surgery. An X-ray of skull (transorbital view) revealed that the electrode array had entered the IAC (**Fig. 5.42**). It may have either been mispositioned during a previous surgery or

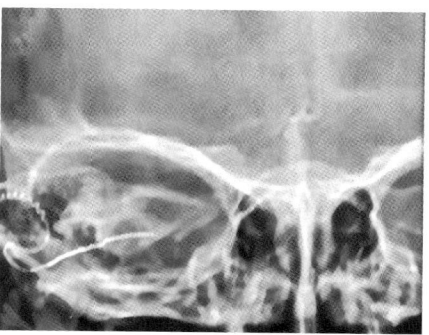

Fig. 5.42 Postoperative X-ray of skull (transorbital view) showing misplaced electrode in the internal auditory canal (IAC).

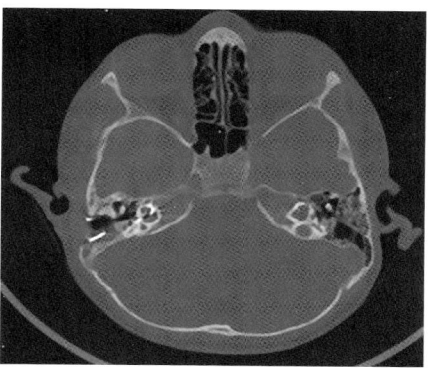

Fig. 5.43 Postoperative high-resolution computed tomography (HRCT) of temporal bone showing the electrode in the basal turn of the cochlea.

may have migrated later into the IAC. As a result, the patient had to be taken for surgical re-exploration, and the implant had to be taken out. Following this, a new implant was placed by bending the electrode in the same way to align with the lateral wall of the basal turn of the cochlea. Post-surgery, HRCT of the temporal bone was taken to ensure the correct placement of the electrode (**Fig. 5.43**). The remaining patients did not face any complication of electrode malposition.

Complete insertion of the electrode array was achieved in all eight patients. CSF gusher was encountered in all cases intraoperatively, and 30-degree head-up position (reverse

Trendelenburg) was given immediately. We waited for 20 minutes for CSF gusher to slow down after which the electrode array was inserted. Firm packing around the electrode with periosteum was the key step to control the CSF gusher. None of the cases needed application of tissue glue or placement of the lumbar drain.

Postoperatively, the patients were prescribed tablet acetazolamide (20 mg/kg/day), laxatives, and antibiotics. They were placed in head-up position and complete bed rest was advised for 5 days postoperatively. No postoperative complications of CSF otorhinorrhea, meningitis, facial paralysis, or vertigo were encountered.

Challenges Experienced

The three most difficult challenges faced were:
- Facial nerve injury.
- CSF gusher.
- Counseling for audiological outcomes:
  - An IP-III deformity is one of the rarest IEMs having X-linked inheritance. It is associated with congenital mixed hearing loss and a fixed stapes footplate. Numerous intraoperative risks associated with this deformity make it a challenge for cochlear implant surgeons.
  - Malposition of electrode array during surgery and migration of electrode during postoperative period occur commonly into the IAC due to wide communication between the cochlea and IAC in IP-III deformity. Few centers advocate the use of intraoperative fluoroscopy to guide the entry of electrode and three-dimensional volume tomography

(3D-VT)–based navigation to perform cochleostomy. We recommended opening a large cochleostomy for easier sealing of round window with soft tissue for management of CSF gusher. Usage of lumbar drain to control CSF gusher is controversial due to risk of postoperative infection. However, the lumbar drain should be opened before the cochleostomy, and it should remain open for 3 days after the surgery.

– In our opinion, good packing of round window opening coupled with conservative measures like bed rest and head end elevation in postoperative period are important steps in management of CSF gusher.

– Selection of the electrode type is important not only to ensure correct insertion of electrode but also to achieve desired audiological outcomes. The number of spiral ganglion cells may be sufficient in IP-III, but the location of neural tissue within the cochlea is divergent. Since modiolus is absent in IP-III, the use of full band circumferentially stimulating electrodes are advocated. Cork electrode, with a "cork" type stopper (25-mm standard electrode), helps in controlling CSF gusher by sealing the cochleostomy.

IP-III is the most challenging as the surgeon faces CSF gush with abnormally placed facial nerve. Knowing your scans preoperatively helps in intraoperative preparation.

References

1. Nance WE, Setleff R, McLeod A, Sweeney A, Cooper C, McConnell F. X-linked mixed deafness with congenital fixation of the stapedial footplate and perilymphatic gusher. Birth Defects Orig Artic Ser 1971;07(4):64–69

2. de Kok YJ, van der Maarel SM, Bitner-Glindzicz M, et al. Association between X-linked mixed deafness and mutations

in the POU domain gene POU3F4. Science 1995;267(5198): 685–688

3. Sennaroglu L, Sarac S, Ergin T. Surgical results of cochlear implantation in malformed cochlea. Otol Neurotol 2006; 27(5):615–623

6 Cochlear Hypoplasia

Introduction

Earlier it was considered that cochlea with 1.5 turns was incomplete partition II (IP-II). When Sennaroglu classified cochlear hypoplasia, the definition of cochlea with 1.5 turns was merged with cochlear hypoplasia.

- External dimensions of those with cochlear hypoplasia are less than those of normal cochlea.
- Internal architecture deformities are present.
- In cochlear hypoplasia, cochlear nerve, cochlear canal, internal auditory canal (IAC), vestibular aqueduct, vestibule, and semicircular canal could be normal/absent/deformed.
- It is of utmost importance to differentiate cochlear hypoplasia on imaging:
  - To know complication that can occur intraoperatively.
  - To choose the choice of electrode for reducing cochlear damage, preserving residual hearing, and for favorable postoperative outcome.

- Sennaroglu classified cochlear hypoplasia into three subtypes in 2010. The subtype IV was added in 2016.
- Development arrest occurring during the 6th week of gestation leads to cochlear hypoplasia I to cochlear hypoplasia III. Arrest happening in between the 10th and 28th weeks of gestation leads to cochlear hypoplasia IV.

Cochlear Hypoplasia Type I

The cochlea is underdeveloped and appears like a small bud, round or ovoid in shape, connected to the IAC. (Note rudimentary otocyst also appears like small bud but never arises from the IAC. Also, rudimentary otocyst does not have a well-developed vestibule.) It lacks modiolus and septa (**Fig. 6.1, Fig. 6.2, Fig. 6.3, Fig. 6.4,** and **Fig. 6.5**).

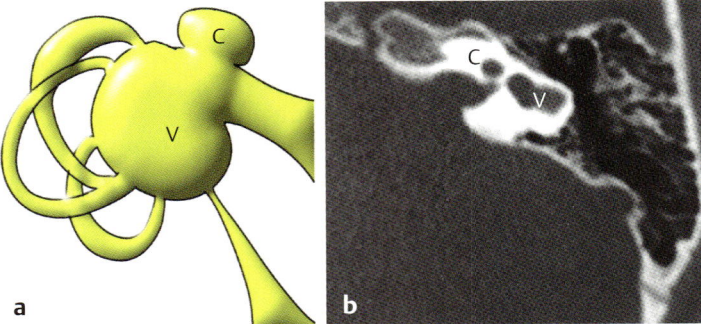

Fig. 6.1 **(a)** Schematic picture showing the cochlea appearing like a bud in cochlear hypoplasia type I (CH-I). **(b)** High-resolution computed tomography (HRCT) of temporal bone axial section showing the bud-like cochlea (C) and vestibule (V).

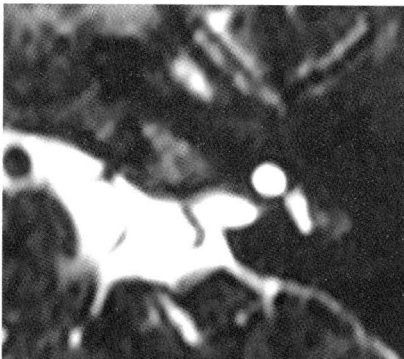

Fig. 6.2 Magnetic resonance imaging (MRI) T2 scan of temporal lobe showing bright illumination corresponding to the computed tomography (CT) picture in **Fig. 6.1**.

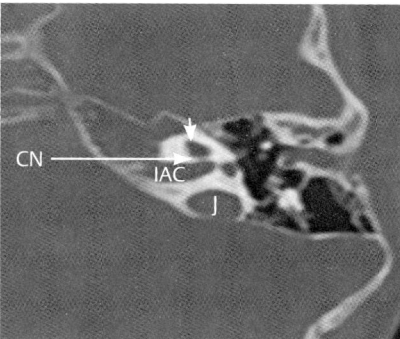

Fig. 6.3 High-resolution computed tomography (HRCT) of temporal bone axial section of left ear showing triangular bud-like cochlea (*white arrow*), internal auditory canal (IAC), cochlear nerve (CN), and jugular bulb (J).

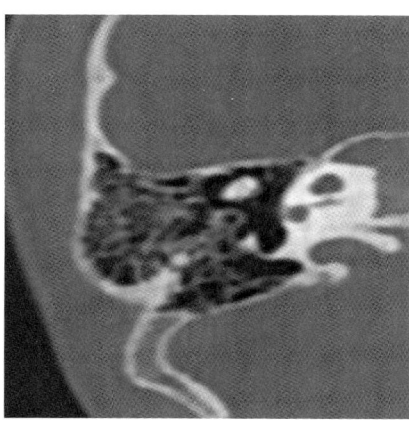

Fig. 6.4 High-resolution computed tomography (HRCT) of temporal bone axial section image of right side with anotia and bulb-like cochlear swelling, but the internal auditory canal (IAC) is not developed resulting in the lack of 7th and 8th nerves. This patient had right side lower motor neuron facial palsy since birth.

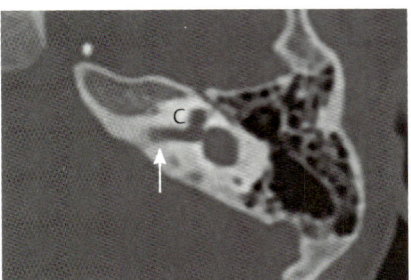

Fig. 6.5 High-resolution computed tomography (HRCT) of temporal bone axial section showing bud-like cochlea (C) along with narrow internal auditory canal (*white arrow*).

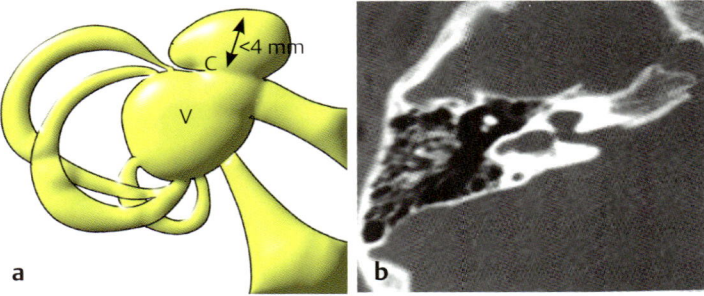

Fig. 6.6 **(a)** Schematic diagram of cochlear hypoplasia type II showing cystic cochlea, dilated vestibule, and vestibular aqueduct; semicircular canal may be underdeveloped. **(b)** High-resolution computed tomography (HRCT) of temporal bone showing cystic swelling arising from the internal auditory canal and dilated vestibule.

Cochlear Hypoplasia Type II

- Cochlea is cystic with deformed modiolus and septa. It looks similar to IP-I. CH-II may also have dilated vestibule and enlarged vestibular aqueduct (**Fig. 6.6, Fig. 6.7, Fig. 6.8, Fig. 6.9, Fig. 6.10, Fig. 6.11, Fig. 6.12,** and **Fig. 6.13**).
- CSF gusher can occur.
- Misplacement of electrode into the IAC can occur.

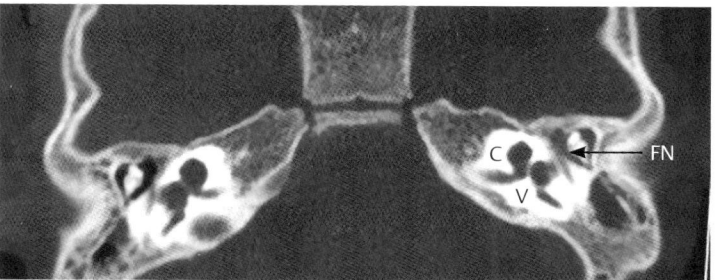

Fig. 6.7 High-resolution computed tomography (HRCT) of temporal bone showing bilateral cochlear hypoplasia type II.

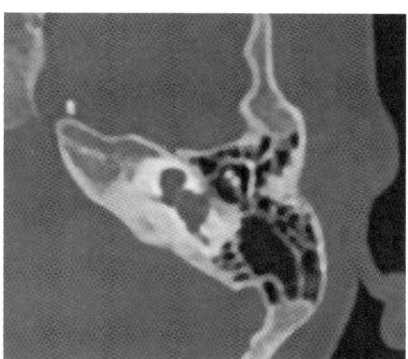

Fig. 6.8 High-resolution computed tomography (HRCT) axial section of temporal bone showing cochlear hypoplasia type II (CH-II) on left side.

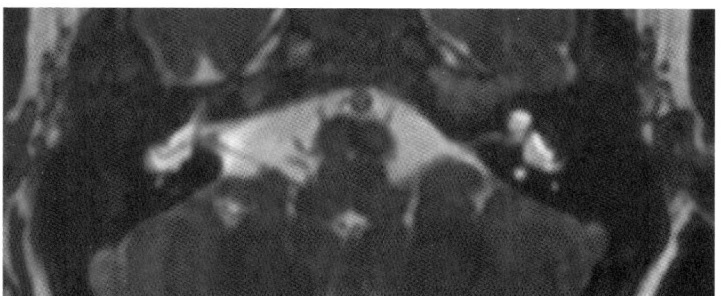

Fig. 6.9 Magnetic resonance imaging (MRI) T2-weighted image showing common cavity on right side and cochlear hypoplasia type II (CH-II) on left side.

101

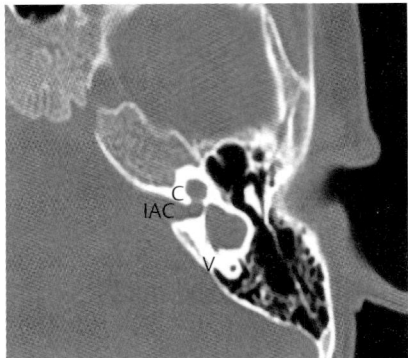

Fig. 6.10 High-resolution computed tomography (HRCT) of temporal bone axial section showing cochlear hypoplasia type II (CH-II) with dilated vestibule and narrow internal auditory canal (IAC).

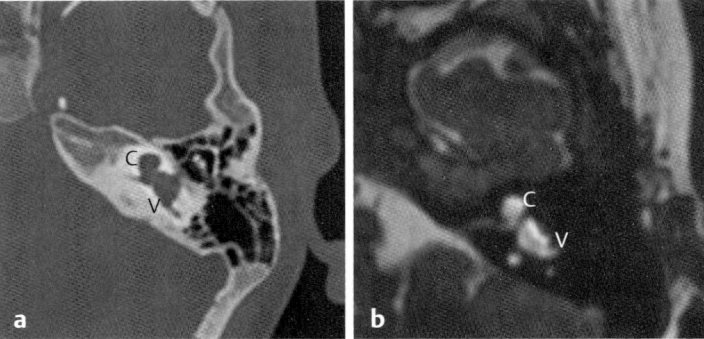

Fig. 6.11 **(a)** Computed tomography (CT) axial section of temporal bone showing cochlear hypoplasia type II with cystic cochlea (C) and dilated vestibule (V). **(b)** Axial magnetic resonance imaging (MRI) T2 sequence of the same patient showing cystic cochlea and loss of modiolus.

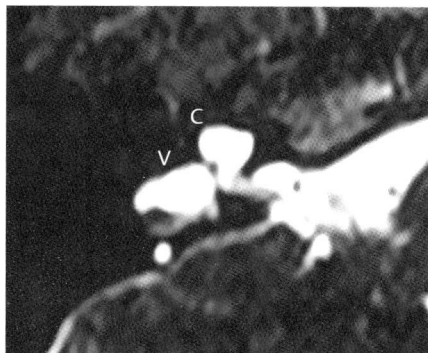

Fig. 6.12 T2-weighted magnetic resonance imaging (MRI) axial section showing cochlear hypoplasia type II (CH-II).

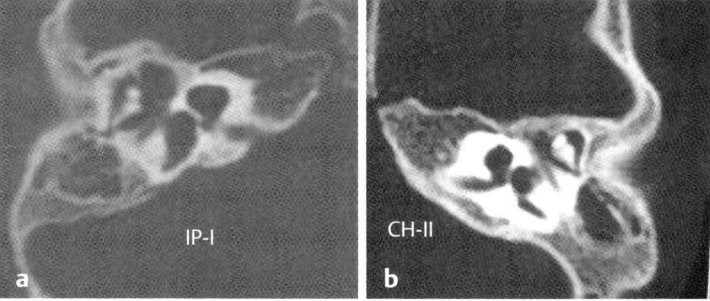

Fig. 6.13 **(a)** High-resolution computed tomography (HRCT) of temporal bone axial section of right side showing cystic cochlea of normal size with dilated vestibule. **(b)** HRCT of temporal bone axial section of left side showing cochlear hypoplasia with cystic cochlea and vestibular dilation.

Cochlear Hypoplasia Type III

- Cochlea looks normal.
- Turns are less than or equal to 1.5 (**Fig. 6.14** and **Fig. 6.15**).

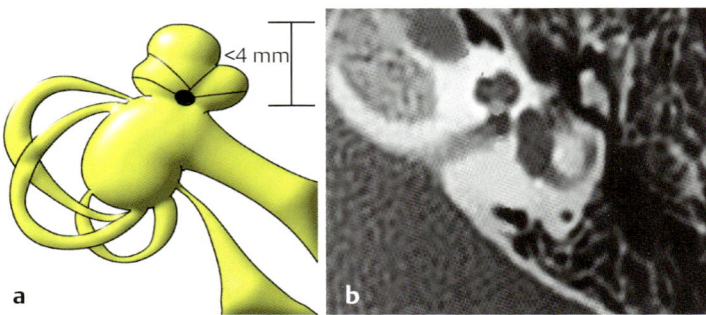

Fig. 6.14 **(a)** Schematic diagram of inner ear showing cochlea with the outer appearance of cochlea similar to that of normal cochlea with modiolus and septa present. **(b)** High-resolution computed tomography (HRCT) of temporal bone axial section showing cochlear hypoplasia type III, with modiolus and septa present.

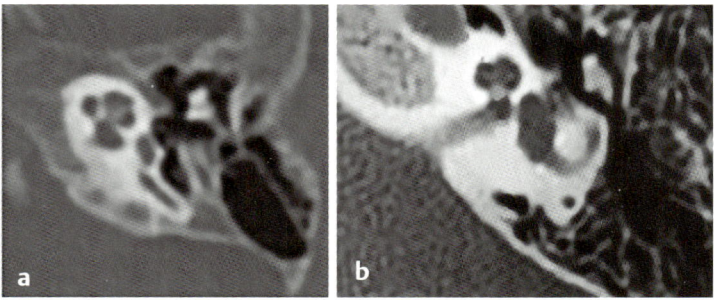

Fig. 6.15 **(a)** High-resolution computed tomography (HRCT) of temporal bone axial section showing normal cochlea with middle and apical turns with modiolus and septa. **(b)** Cochlear hypoplasia type III with modiolus and septa but height less than 4 mm.

Cochlear Hypoplasia Type IV

- Normal basal turn.
- Hypoplastic middle and apical turn (**Fig. 6.16**).

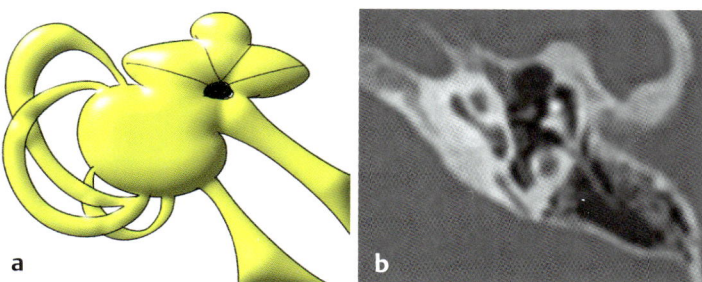

Fig. 6.16 **(a)** Schematic diagram of cochlear hypoplasia type IV showing normal basal turn but hypoplastic apical and middle turn. **(b)** High-resolution computed tomography (HRCT) of temporal bone axial section showing the basal turn is normal, and apical and middle turns are hypoplastic and located anteromedial to basal turn rather than in central part.

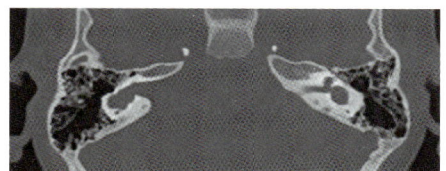

Fig. 6.17 High-resolution computed tomography (HRCT) of temporal bone axial section showing common cavity on right side and cochlear hypoplasia type I (CH-I) on left side.

Cases of Malformations

Surgeon should be cautious of different anomalies on both sides in one patient. One should rule out presence of tilt. This helps in intra operative planning and post operative complications (**Fig. 6.17**).

Cochlear Hypoplasia

The types of cochlear hypoplasia are described in **Table 6.1**.

Table 6.1 Types of cochlear hypoplasia

Cochlear hypoplasia		Modiolus	Septa
I	Bud	Absent	Absent
II	Cystic	Deformed	Deformed
III	Normal	Short	Reduced
IV	Hypoplastic apical and middle turn	Well formed	Normal

Case 1
Chiari Malformation with CH-IV

Refer **Fig. 6.18, Fig. 6.19, Fig. 6.20,** and **Fig. 6.21**.

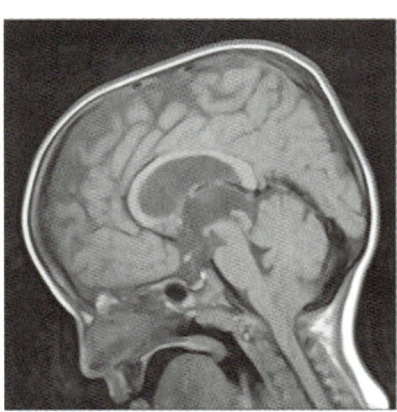

Fig. 6.18 Magnetic resonance imaging (MRI) of brain (T1) mid-sagittal image showing cerebellar tonsil herniating into foramen magnum.

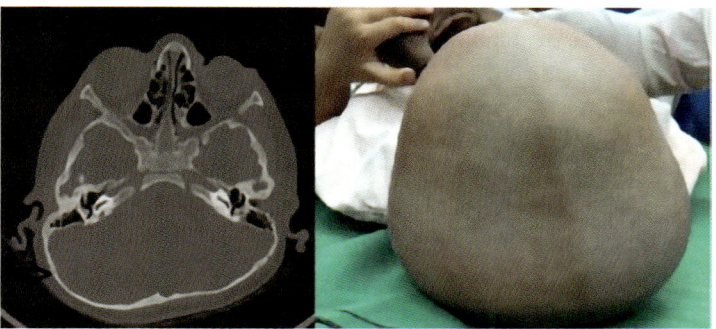

Fig. 6.19 Left hemisphere larger than the right.

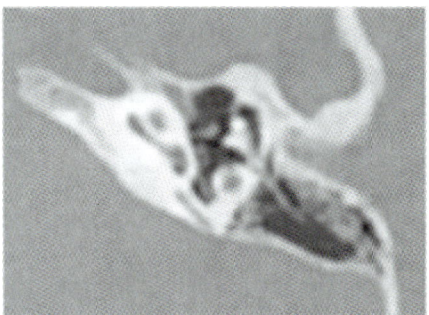

Fig. 6.20 Axial high-resolution computed tomography (HRCT) of temporal bone showing hypoplastic middle and apical turns.

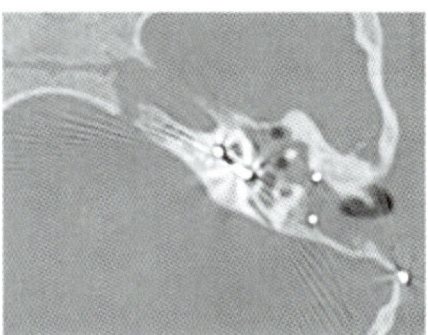

Fig. 6.21 High-resolution computed tomography (HRCT) of temporal bone showing electrode array in cochlea.

7 Cochlear Aperture: Bony Cochlear Nerve Canal

"Wide cochlear aperture—a risk factor for CSF gusher in cochlear implant surgery: often missed & seldom reported in HRCT temporal bone scan."

Introduction

Even a perfectly done cochlear implant by an experienced and skillful surgeon is not exempt from failures, if due precautions are not taken to prevent spread of infection into the intracranial cavity via cochleostomy. It is well established that cerebrospinal fluid (CSF) leak encountered during cochlear implant surgery has to be dealt with utmost seriousness, both intraoperatively and perioperatively, in order to avoid meningitis and implant infection. It is, therefore, imperative to identify potential patients who have a likelihood of CSF leak during surgery. Among the many predictable causes of intraoperative CSF leak, the common ones that have been published in textbooks and peer-reviewed journals are various malformation of the cochlea, like the incomplete partition II (IP-II), incomplete partition III (IP-III), and common cavity malformation. Cochlear aperture (CA) also called as bony canal of cochlear nerve (BCNC) is a transition zone made of fibro-osseus tissue between the CSF containing internal auditory canal (IAC) and the vestibule. There are few studies which have discussed the width of CA beyond a certain dimension as a risk factor for intraoperative CSF leak. This chapter intends to emphasize the importance of identifying this easy-to-miss radiological diagnosis in order to avoid CSF leak (**Fig. 7.1**). Narrow CA is discussed in the chapter 10 on internal acoustic meatus.

Cochlear aperture also known as **modiolar base**, is a fibro-osseus structure at the base of the modiolus that transmits blood vessels and nerve fibers from the spiral

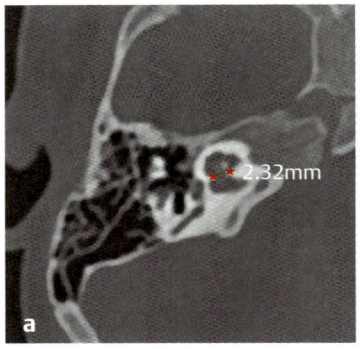
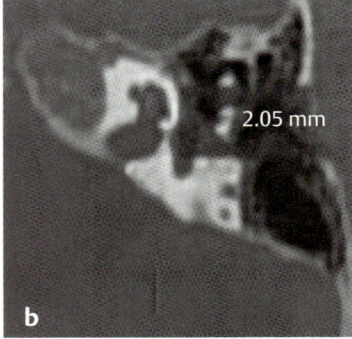

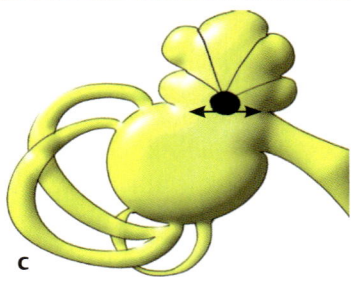

Fig. 7.1 **(a–c)** High-resolution computed tomography (HRCT) of temporal bone showing measurement of cochlear aperture (Dicom viewer software).

ganglion to the cochlear nerve (**Fig. 7.2**). There are three types of CSF presentation during cochlear implant surgery. These are pulsation (no leak, just pulsation), oozers (intermittent, slow to fill up, leak lasting 5–10 minutes), and gushers (profuse, fills up rapidly, pulsating, lasts 15–20 minutes). Among the latter two varieties of CSF leak, (i.e., gushers and oozers), gusher more specifically makes insertion of implant electrode difficult and may cause postoperative meningitis. Therefore, the possibility of a gusher should be diagnosed preoperatively, and necessary precautions should be taken. Overall, the reported incidence of gushers in cochlear implantation is found to be 1%.[1,2] However, it is seen more often in patients with radiologically seen inner ear abnormalities. Furthermore, in cochlear implantation with radiologically known inner ear malformations gushers are seen in about 50% of cases.[3] Nonetheless, there are multiple reports of cases where there were no apparent radiologically reported abnormalities, and yet CSF gusher was encountered during surgery. The oozer phenomenon is mostly due to abnormalities of cochlear aqueduct and vestibular aqueduct, while gusher phenomenon is mostly due to IAC abnormalities.[4]

Although the IAC in different individuals may differ greatly in size, the two canals of any person are identical or

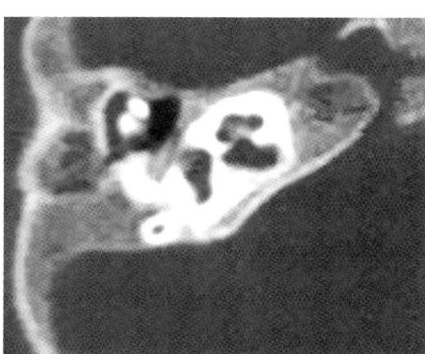

Fig. 7.2 Wide cochlear aperture with otomasto-iditis with forward-lying sigmoid.

111

vary by no more than 1 mm.[4] The medial most part of the cone-shaped modiolus, the base of which plugs in a fashion which cocks the IAC, is called the **lamina cribrosa** (thin fibro-osseus plate). The lamina cribrosa is pierced by the neural structures and blood vessels (originating in most cases from the anterior–inferior cerebellar artery). It has a dural and arachnoid covering medially and forms a barrier between the inner ear and the subarachnoid space.[4] The lamina cribrosa is the most likely site of CSF leakage.[5] The CSF may communicate with fluid around the cochlear nerve in the center of the modiolus and channels into the Rosenthal canal as well as spirally arranged spaces for the anterior and posterior spiral veins.[6] Schuknecht was the first to describe small pores in the scala tympani surface in cats, and he called them **"canaliculi perforantes."**[7] The endosteal layer of scala tympani, although implicated in many studies to be of significance in perilymph hemostasis, is not of sufficient strength to offer resistance to CSF flow from the IAC if the overlying bone is deficient.[3]

The basal turn of cochlea, particularly the scala tympani in this part of the basal turn, is in close proximity to the posterolateral aspect of the IAC. Often the bone is deficient here, providing an easy route for CSF to leak into the scala tympani. Modiolar bone defect has been classified into seven types. It appears that type 6 (subtotal absence of modiolus) and type 7 (complete absence of modiolus) when reviewed on computed tomography (CT) scan will show an apparently wide CA. Wider communication from an enlarged aperture generates larger gradients in hydrostatic pressure between the subarachnoid space and cochlear modiolus, which may lead to CSF gusher. CT can be an important tool in prediction of a gusher. CT is also useful in illustrating other findings which could contribute to the CSF leak. When there is a total bone defect in the modiolar base, it permits all high-pressure CSF in the internal acoustic canal to enter the cochlea; thus, intraoperative CSF leakage increases in severity and leads to a gusher. Yet, if there is a thin plate of bone in the modiolar base, CSF leakage is intermittent and less severe, which are characteristics of oozing.

What to Look for in a CT Scan?

The bony partition between the IAC and the basal turn of the cochlea is much thinner on the lateral posterior aspect when compared to the anteromedial part. However, there is often a failure to notice this defect, and hence preoperatively being discounted as normal CT. It is due to the **"partial volume effect"** (**Fig. 7.3** and **Fig. 7.4**). Categorically speaking, when there is a radiological defect in this lateral posterior aspect of the IAC, it leads to widened CA. The lateral–posterior boundary of CA is this thin ledge of bone (when compared to its medial counterpart) that separates the IAC from the scala tympani of the basal turn of the cochlea. But not all patients with such a defect apparently seen on CT or magnetic resonance imaging will have CSF leaks. This can be because of presence of fibrous

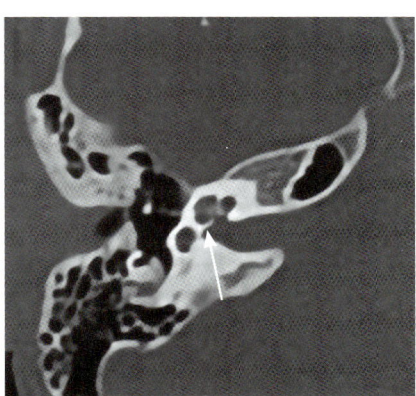

Fig. 7.3 High-resolution computed tomography (HRCT) of right temporal bone showing the normal size cochlear aperture. The posterior lateral bony ledge is highlighted with a *white arrow*.

113

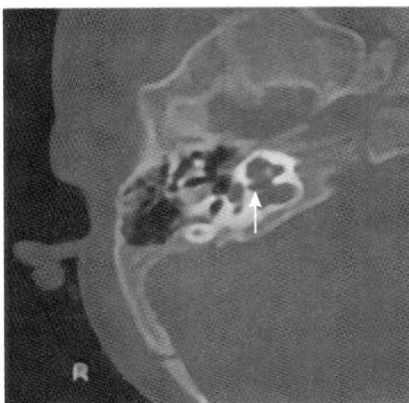

Fig. 7.4 High-resolution computed tomography (HRCT) of right temporal bone with thinned out nearly missing ledge of posterolateral bone, leading to a widened cochlear aperture (*white arrow*).

bands at the junction between the IAC and inner ear, which cannot be seen by presently available imaging techniques.

Normal Dimension of Cochlear Aperture, and it's Significance

At our institute we accept a CA width of 1.9 as normal, and any case with scan having CA of width ≥2.0 mm is reflagged for possibility of CSF gusher. Identification of wide CA has prognostic significance and critical implications in preoperative counseling. Temporal bone imaging plays an important role in identifying inner ear abnormalities, and in systematic review prior to surgery, and including measurement of CA dimension is critical, which is often missed by radiologist due to "partial volume effect." Our recommendation is any CA width of ≥2.0 mm must alert the surgeon of possible CSF leak, and he/she must be prepared to handle intraoperative CSF gusher.

References

1. Sennaroglu L. Histopathology of inner ear malformations: do we have enough evidence to explain pathophysiology? Cochlear Implants Int 2016;17(1):3–20

2. Ding X, Tian H, Wang W, Zhang D. Cochlear implantation in China: review of 1,237 cases with an emphasis on complications. ORL J Otorhinolaryngol Relat Spec 2009;71(4):192–195

3. Sennaroglu L, Sarac S, Ergin T. Surgical results of cochlear implantation in malformed cochlea. Otol Neurotol 2006;27(5):615–623

4. Bajin MD, Pamuk AE, Pamuk G, Özgen B, Sennaroğlu L. The association between modiolar base anomalies and intraoperative cerebrospinal fluid leakage in patients with incomplete partition type-II anomaly: a classification system and presentation of 73 cases. Otol Neurotol 2018;39(7):e538–e542

5. Schuknecht HF. Mondini dysplasia; a clinical and pathological study. Ann Otol Rhinol Laryngol Suppl 1980;89(1 Pt 2):1–23

6. Küçük B, Abe K, Ushiki T, Inuyama Y, Fukuda S, Ishikawa K. Microstructures of the bony modiolus in the human cochlea: a scanning electron microscopic study. J Electron Microsc (Tokyo) 1991;40(3):193–197

7. Schuknecht HF, Seifi AE. Experimental observations on the fluid physiology of the inner ear. Ann Otol Rhinol Laryngol 1963;72:687–712

8 Vestibular and Cochlear Aqueduct

Vestibular Aqueduct

- **Valvassori and Clemis criteria:** If the width of the vestibular aqueduct (VA) is more than 1.5 mm, when measured at the midpoint of a line joining its course from the posterior cranial fossa opening to vestibule, it is defined as enlarged vestibular aqueduct (EVA) (**Fig. 8.1** and **Fig. 8.2**).

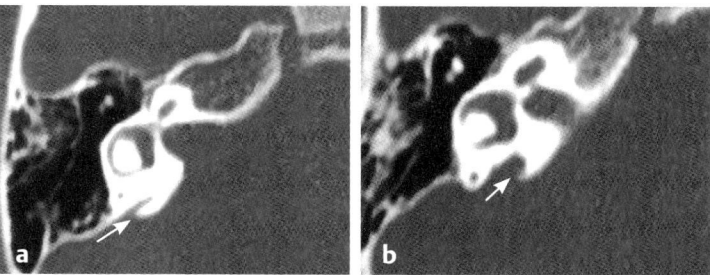

Fig. 8.1 **(a)** High-resolution computed tomography (HRCT) of temporal bone axial section showing vestibular aqueduct (*white arrow*). **(b)** HRCT of temporal bone axial section showing enlarged vestibular aqueduct according to Valvassori and Clemis criteria (*white arrow*).

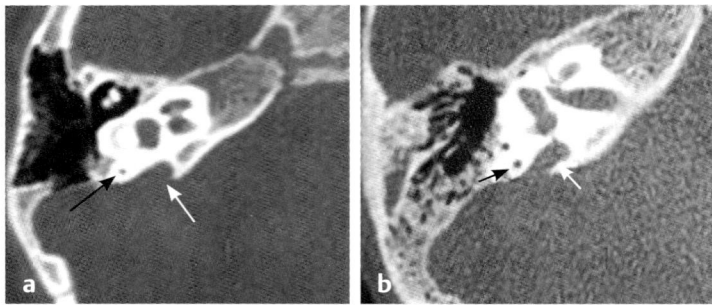

Fig. 8.2 (a, b) Enlarged vestibular aqueduct (EVA) according to Wilson criteria (*white arrow* shows EVA, *black arrow* shows posterior semicircular canal [SCC]).

- **Wilson criteria (Fig. 8.2):** If any segment of VA is twice that of the adjacent posterior semicircular canal, it is defined as EVA.

Cochlear Aqueduct

- Cochlear aqueduct is a bony canal connecting sub-arachnoid space to the basal turn of cochlea.
- It surrounds the perilymphatic duct.
- On axial computed tomography (CT) scan, cochlear aqueduct can be divided into four segments (**Fig. 8.3** and **Fig. 8.4**):
  - Lateral orifice (LO): Opening into the basal turn of cochlea.
  - Otic capsule (OC): Lateral orifice opens here (through labyrinthine bone).
  - Petrous apex (PA): Otic capsule opens here (comes through bone which may be pneumatized or filled with marrow).

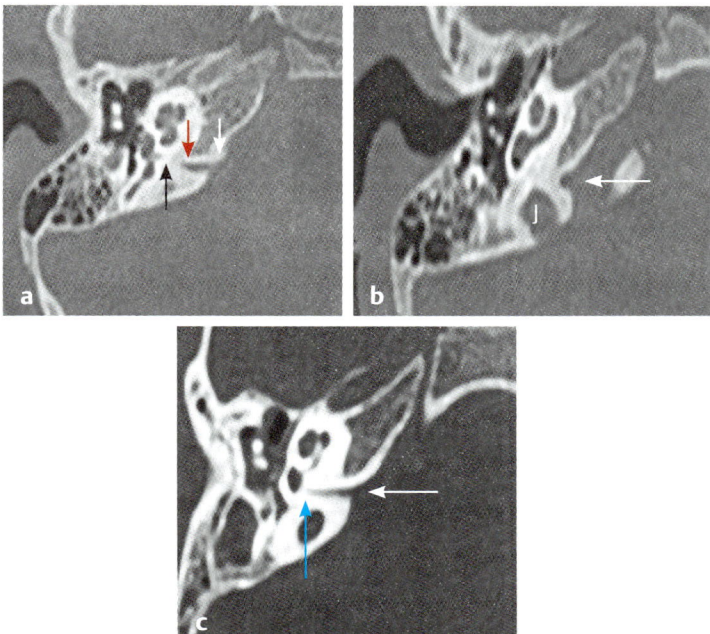

Fig. 8.3 **(a)** High-resolution computed tomography (HRCT) of temporal bone axial section showing medial orifice (*white arrow*), otic capsule (*red arrow*), and petrous apex segment (*black arrow*). **(b)** HRCT of temporal bone axial section showing medial orifice (*white arrow*) and jugular bulb (J). **(c)** HRCT of temporal bone axial section showing patent cochlear aqueduct with medial orifice (*white arrow*) and lateral orifice (*blue arrow*).

 – Medial orifice (MO): Petrous apex opens into subarachnoid space in a funnel-shaped medial orifice.
    ○ Lateral orifice, otic capsule, and petrous apex are not visualized in high percentage of CT scans.
    ○ Medial orifice is the most visible portion on the CT scan.

119

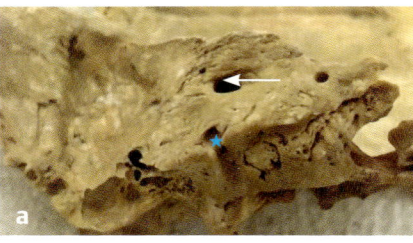

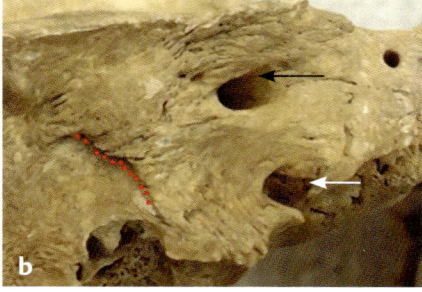

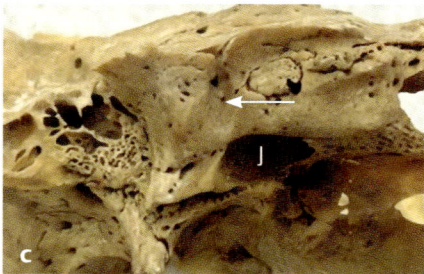

Fig. 8.4 **(a)** Temporal bone image showing internal auditory canal (*white arrow*) and opening for cochlear canaliculus (*blue star*). **(b)** Temporal bone image showing internal auditory canal (*black arrow*), opening for cochlear canaliculus (*white arrow*), and opening for vestibular canaliculus (*red dots*). **(c)** Temporal bone image showing jugular bulb (J) and incomplete bone covering over the petrosal fossa (*white arrow*).

- Medial orifice opens into anterior division of jugular foramen, close to glossopharyngeal nerve below the internal auditory canal.
- Diameter of the cochlear aqueduct is inconsistent.

Embryology

Embryology explains enlarged or patent aqueduct may or may not be associated with inner ear malformations due to separate embryological origin of cochlear aqueduct (forms in mesoderm of perilymphatic duct) and membranous labyrinth (forms in otic capsule).

Conclusion

- Cochlear aqueduct act as route of transmission of bacterial infection between the subarachnoid space and the perilymph within the inner ear.
- Cerebrospinal fluid (CSF) gusher can occur as a result of increased inner ear pressure.
- Perilymph fistulas can occur due to defects in the bony portion of the fundus of the internal auditory canal.
- Inner ear pressure is maintained by the bony capsule, round window, and oval window.

Note: Cochlear aqueduct is considered to be insignificant, but it is a distinct entity leading to CSF gusher in CT scan reported to be normal.

Suggested Reading

Jackler RK, Hwang PH. Enlargement of the cochlear aqueduct: fact or fiction? Otolaryngol Head Neck Surg 1993;109(1):14–25

Rask-Andersen H, Stahle J, Wilbrand H. Human cochlear aqueduct and its accessory canals. Ann Otol Rhinol Laryngol Suppl 1977;86(5 Pt 2 Suppl 42):1–16

9 Cochlear Ossification

Introduction

- Cochlear ossification appears to be the result of inflammatory processes within perilymphatic spaces of cochlea. It is a pathological condition characterized by neo-ossification (new bone formation).
- It can spread through the following routes:
  – Tympanogenic (meningitidis).
  – Meningogenic.
  – Hematogenous.

- The pathogens involved are *S. pneumonia*, neisseria meningitidis (N.), and *H. influenzae*.
- Infection in the subarachnoid space reaches the cochlea via cochlear aqueduct (link between cerebrospinal fluid to inner ear).
- The etiological factors are as follows:
  – Otosclerosis.
  – Inflammation.
  – Trauma.
  – Ototoxic medication.
  – Leukemia.

- Temporal bone tumor.
- Autoimmune disease.
- Labyrinthine artery occlusion.

Process of Ossification

The process of ossification is described in **Flowchart 9.1**.

- It starts and is mostly confined to the round window and proximal scala tympani. It may then progress within cochlear lumen causing partial or complete obliteration.
- The occurrence and degree of ossification is related to imaging modality, causative pathogen, age at disease, and time between infection and imaging.

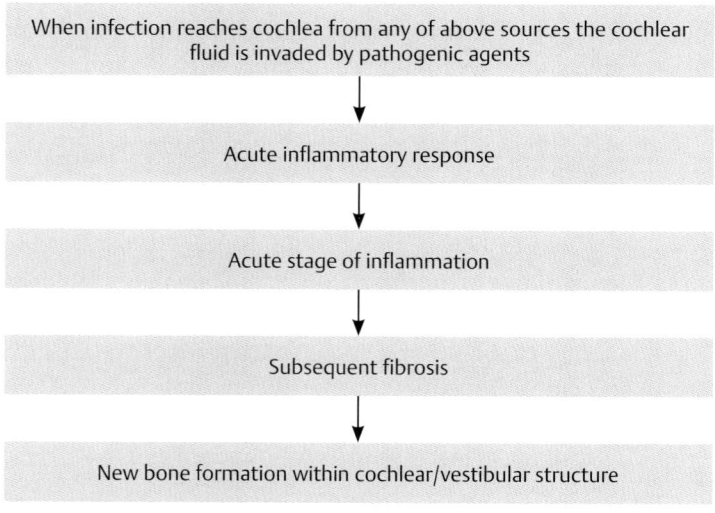

Flowchart 9.1 Process of ossification.

Imaging Techniques

- Computed tomography (CT) has a high specificity in diagnosing bone tissue pathologies. CT scan shows labyrinthine calcification processes earlier than magnetic resonance imaging (MRI). MRI (T2-weighted images) is sensitive for fluid and more sensitive for formation of fibrosis-induced signal intensity of the labyrinthine structures.
- Cochlear ossification remains a challenge in cochlear implantation.
- The extent and location of ossification have implication on the choice of surgical approaches, cochlear drilling, and electrode.
- The surgeon should be prepared for modification of the following:
  - Surgical techniques.
  - Choice of arrays.
  - Extent of drilling—round window, basal turn, middle turn, or drill out.
  - Scala tympani or scala vestibule insertion.
  - Partial or complete insertion.
  - Complications: Cerebrospinal fluid gusher, first tract in superior semicircular canal or in carotid, facial nerve stimulation.
- Postoperative imaging is of vital importance in cases of cochlear implantation and ossification (**Fig. 9.1, Fig. 9.2,** and **Fig. 9.3**).

125

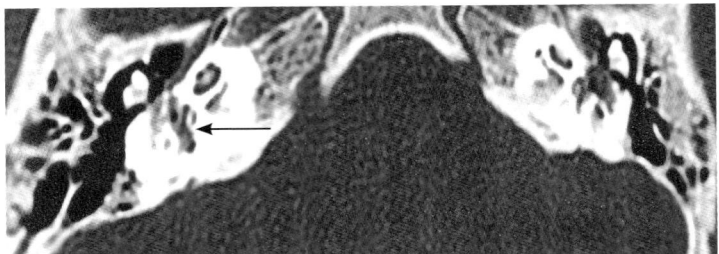

Fig. 9.1 Computed tomography (CT) axial section of petrous part of temporal bone showing round window ossification (*black arrow*).

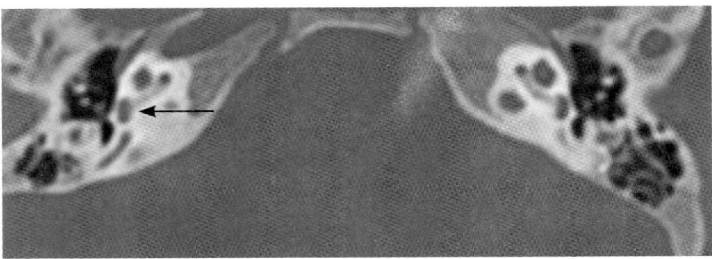

Fig. 9.2 High-resolution computed tomography (HRCT) axial section of petrous temporal bone showing partial ossification of basal turn of cochlea (*black arrow*).

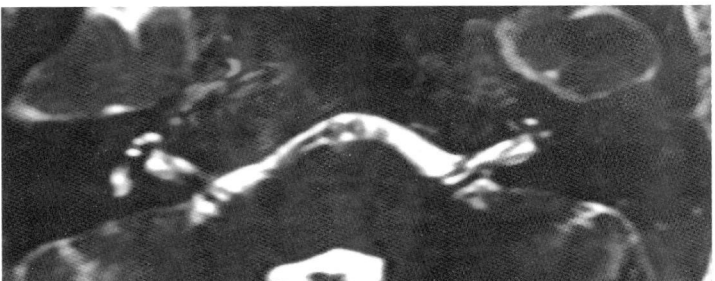

Fig. 9.3 Inner ear fluid: T2-weighted magnetic resonance imaging (MRI) axial section showing partial extinction of the T2 hyperintensity of the endolymph of both the cochlea.

Case 1

A case of leukemia and chronic suppurative otitis media (CSOM).

- Source of infection was tympanogenic and hematogenous.
- **Fig. 9.4(a–e)** and **Fig. 9.5** show series of axial high-resolution computed tomography (HRCT) of temporal bone.

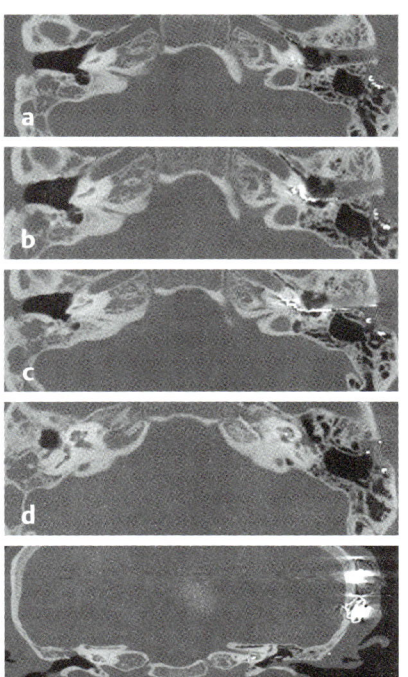

Fig. 9.4 **(a–d)** Ossification of all turns of cochlea on right side. Left side electrode array seen going to basal turn of cochlea and with incomplete insertion. **(e)** Coronal section showing electrode array in situ on left side.

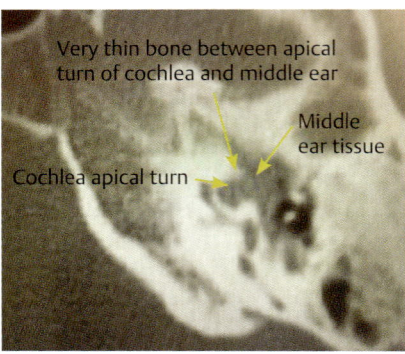

Very thin bone between apical turn of cochlea and middle ear

Middle ear tissue

Cochlea apical turn

Fig. 9.5 High-resolution computed tomography (HRCT) of temporal bone axial section showing sclerosis extending into cochlea.

Tympanogenic Labyrinthine Ossificans

Ossification is an emergency in hearing impaired kids.

Introduction

Labyrinthine obliterans is defined as a condition of membranous labyrinth where the labyrinthine structures get sclerosed because of inflammatory response. When there is new bone formation along with sclerosis it is called labyrinthine ossificans. There are numerous factors which initiate the inflammatory process in the inner ear. One among the many factors is the spread of infection from the middle ear cleft, resulting in tympanogenic labyrinthine sclerosis. Other causes include autoimmune conditions of the inner ear, meningogenic or hematogenous spread of infection, sickle cell anemia, leukemia, post rubella vaccination, otosclerosis, and traumatic and postsurgical inflammatory response. Although rare, inflammatory or granulomatous diseases can also mimic or present as labyrinthine sclerosis. The patient often presents with sensorineural hearing loss and/or vertigo.

Acute otitis media (AOM) is a very common condition in the pediatric age group, which at times can progress to chronicity. In this era of antibiotics, the complications of AOM or chronic otitis media (COM) are seen less often, and they mostly occur in immunocompromised patients. The complications and sequalae of the AOM are many and are classified as intracranial and extracranial. The extracranial complications are further divided into intratemporal and extratemporal. Here we present a case of otitis media which resulted in facial palsy and bilateral labyrinthine sclerosis.

Case Report

A 2 years and 3 months old child was presented to our outpatient department for evaluation with complaint of delayed speech and decreased hearing. On detailed history taking and evaluation, we noticed that the child had undergone multiple radiological imaging and surgical interventions at various other hospitals. The brief history of events is given in the following in chronological order. The radiological findings are summarized in **Table 9.1**.

At the age of 9 months, the child had an episode of right ear discharge of sudden onset associated with lower motor neuron (LMN) type of facial palsy on the same side (Grade III House-Brackmann grading). The same was managed with short tapering course of corticosteroids and intravenous antibiotics.

At the age of 10 months, the child continued to have ear discharge with no obvious LMN facial palsy, but she developed right postauricular abscess with no signs and symptoms of intracranial extension and onset of left ear discharge.

At the age of 12 months, the child continued to have ear discharge despite being under broad-spectrum antibiotic therapy. Examination under microscope showed presence of granulation tissue with discharge in the external auditory canal. Culture and sensitivity of right ear discharge showed

129

Table 9.1 Series of scans done at different months

Age at the time of investigation	Type of imaging	Summary of the findings	Images
9 months	1.5T MRI	Features suggestive of old ischemic lesions in parietal lobe in periventricular deep white matter on either side.	
10 months	HRCT of temporal bone	Soft tissue density areas seen in bilateral middle ear cavity. Normal ossicles on either side. Small abscess in subcutaneous plane in right postauricular region. Normal cochlea and semicircular canals.	

Age at the time of investigation	Type of imaging	Summary of the findings	Images
12 months	HRCT of temporal bone	Right ear—ill-defined soft tissue density areas with internal fluid collection involving external ear, hypo-meso-epitympanum. Erosion of scutum, anterior process of malleus, incus, and stapes suprastructure, floor of tympanic segment of facial nerve, pyramidal eminence, cochlear eminence. Medial erosion of cochlea and vestibule with involvement of posterior and lateral semicircular canals. Lateral erosion of mastoid. Left ear—ill-defined soft tissue density areas with internal fluid collection involving external ear, hypo-meso-epitympanum. Erosion of scutum, anterior process of malleus, incus, and stapes suprastructure, nerve, pyramidal eminence, cochlear eminence. Medial erosion of cochlea and vestibule with involvement of posterior and lateral semicircular canals. Petrous apex, internal auditory canal, and facial canal normal.	

(Continued)

Table 9.1 (*Continued*) Series of scans done at different months

Age at the time of investigation	Type of imaging	Summary of the findings	Images
12 months	1.5T MRI with contrast	The soft tissue densities in HRCT demonstrated hyperintense signals on T2-weighted and FLAIR images. On DW images no evidence of significant effusion restriction is noted. Postcontrast soft tissue showed homogenous intense enhancement	

Age at the time of investigation	Type of imaging	Summary of the findings	Images
1 year and 4 months	HRCT of temporal bone	Compared with HRCT at 12 months, there was evidence of rapidly progressive, bilateral, diffuse, confluent, concentric pericochlear, cochlear, and vestibular sclerosis, which replaced the lucency around the otic capsule. There is complete obliteration of right otic capsule and near-complete obliteration of left otic capsule.	

(Continued)

Table 9.1 (*Continued*) Series of scans done at different months

Age at the time of investigation	Type of imaging	Summary of the findings	Images
1 year and 4 months	1.5T MRI with contrast	The soft tissues in external canal showed T2 hyperintensity and DW images showed no restriction of diffusion. On 3D fast imaging employing steady state acquisition (FIESTA), there is obliteration of high fluid spaces of membranous labyrinth. Postcontrast T1 images revealed mild enhancement of the right apical turn of cochlea and middle and apical turn on left side. Vestibule and SCC are unremarkable bilaterally. Internal auditory canal and petrous apex appear normal. Normal thickness of cochlear nerves bilaterally.	

Age at the time of investigation	Type of imaging	Summary of the findings	Images
2 years and 3 months	HRCT of temporal bone	Absence of cochlear turns, hypoplastic semicircular canals and vestibule, narrow internal auditory canal, and changes of otomastoiditis bilaterally.	

(Continued)

Table 9.1 (*Continued*) Series of scans done at different months

Age at the time of investigation	Type of imaging	Summary of the findings	Images
2 years and 3 months	1.5T MRI with contrast	Nonvisualization of cochlea, vestibule, and semicircular canals on either side. VIIth and VIIIth cranial nerves within internal auditory canal visualized and symmetrical bilaterally. Small hyperintense foci in bilateral frontoparietal periventricular white matter.	

Abbreviations: DW, diffusion-weighted; FIESTA; FLAIR, fluid-attenuated inversion recovery; HRCT, high-resolution computed tomography; MRI, magnetic resonance imaging; SCC, semicircular canal.

the presence of *Pseudomonas* species and methicillin-resistant staphylococci species sensitive to piperacillin–tazobactam and ceftazidime. The patient at this stage was treated with piperacillin tazobactam intravenously with dosage adjustments as per the age and weight.

At the age of 1 year and 1 month, the child continued to have ear discharge but was symptomatically better than before. A biopsy of the external canal granulation tissue was performed, and the histopathological report showed signs of chronic osteomyelitis with negative immunohistochemical markers for Langerhans histiocytosis.

At the age of 1 year and 5 months, the child underwent left side mastoid exploration at an outside center. Intraoperative findings showed presence of extensive granulation tissues in the middle ear cleft with erosion of all the three ossicles with nonvisualization of the foot plate of stapes. The histopathological examination report of the middle ear tissue showed a picture of active on chronic inflammation with no presence of acid-fast bacilli on Ziehl staining and cartridge based nucleic acid amplification test (CB-NAAT) (**Fig. 9.6**). The child's ear became dry after the procedure for a period of 4 months.

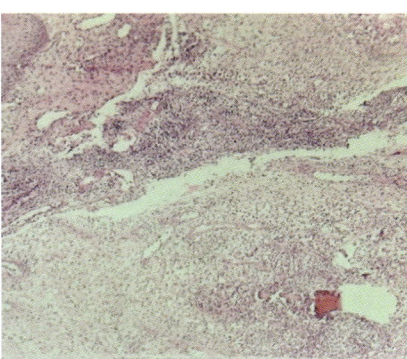

Fig. 9.6 Histopathology image of middle ear mucosa showing signs of acute on chronic inflammation with no granuloma.

The child's hearing sensitivity started deteriorating significantly, which made the patient's parents to seek intervention at our center which is a designated center of implant surgery. The child presented to our outpatient department (OPD) 8 months after the left mastoid exploration surgery. At the time of presentation, the child was active, playful, not responding to simple commands due to lack of localization of sound, and absent speech. On examination, the right ear showed granulation tissue inside the external auditory canal with minimal ear discharge, nonvisualization of tympanic membrane, and normal facial nerve function. Left side showed postoperative canal wall up surgery with minimal discharge and neotympanic membrane residual perforation and clinically normal facial nerve function. After a complete clinical, audiological, and radiological evaluation, the child was found to have severe to profound hearing loss with complete obliteration of bilateral membranous labyrinth with intact cochlear nerve.

Conclusion

The inflammatory agents from the middle ear can enter the labyrinth via hematogenous route, bony canals, or directly through the round or oval window. Regardless of the etiological agent, the inner ear inflammatory process follows a similar pattern, starting with stage of inflammation followed by stage of fibrosis and finally stage of ossification. The various stages can co-exist at the same time in the different areas of the inner ear. It has been found that maximum ossification occurs toward the basal part of cochlea near the round window. Early intervention is of utmost importance in these cases as the success of cochlear implant depends on the extent of ossification. Complete ossification may preclude or make cochlear implant difficult or indicate brain stem implants.

CT scan is believed to be more specific in identifying new bone formation but not sensitive in initial stages of the inner ear inflammatory reaction. In such cases the use of MRI is very helpful. The increase in density or haziness of the inner ear fluid space gives an indication of fibroblastic proliferative stage in T2 images with contrast.

Suggested Reading

Mattiola LR, Makowiecky M, Salles CEG, Cardoso MP, Cahali S. Labyrinthitis ossificans. Report of one case and literature review. Int Arch Otorhinol 2008;12(2):300–302

Page N, Kearns D. Radiology quiz case 2. Labyrinthitis ossificans secondary to suppurative labyrinthitis. Arch Otolaryngol Head Neck Surg 2011;137(3):303–305, 305

Thind RK, Ho GC, Yap D, Hunt A. 508 The early use of intratympanic steroid injections in the treatment of labyrinthitis obliterans—a case report. Br J Surg 2021;108(Suppl_6):znab259.295

10 Internal Acoustic Meatus

Introduction

- The internal auditory canal (IAC) is a bony canal which is 2 to 8 mm wide and passes through petrous part of the temporal bone.
- It lies between the cerebellopontine angle and labyrinth.
- Facial nerve and vestibulocochlear nerve get transmitted via the IAC.
- The vestibulocochlear nerve divides into the following branches:
  - Cochlear nerve.
  - Superior vestibular nerve.
  - Inferior vestibular nerve.

- Facial nerve and cochlear nerve occupy the antero-superior and anteroinferior compartment, respectively, in the IAC divided by the falciform crest (horizontally).
- Superior vestibular nerve and inferior vestibular nerve lie in posterosuperior and posteroinferior compartment.

Abnormalities of Internal Auditory Canal

- On computed tomography (CT) scan, the IAC is evaluated in axial section by measuring the width at the center of the canal.
- Normal diameter is 2 to 8 mm.
  - If less than 2 mm it is termed as stenotic (**Fig. 10.1**).
  - If ≥8 mm it is termed as dilated.

- The IAC is measured to assess the presence of cochlear nerve (**Fig. 10.2**). If dilated, other cochlear anomalies should be ruled out to assess for cerebrospinal fluid gusher intraoperatively (**Fig. 10.3**).
- Measurement of the IAC alone is not sufficient to assess the deficiency of cochlear nerve.

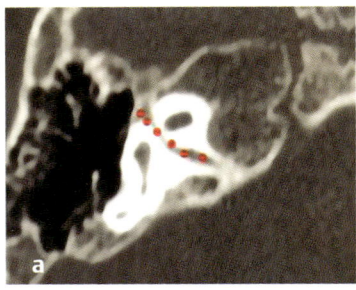
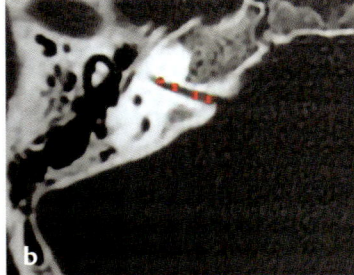
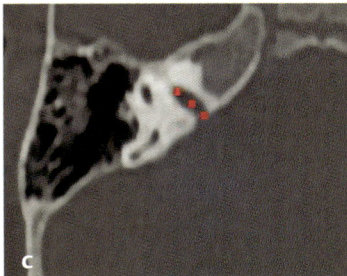

Fig. 10.1 **(a–c)** Axial high-resolution computed tomography (HRCT) of temporal bone showing stenotic internal auditory canal with only facial nerve in canal (*red dots*).

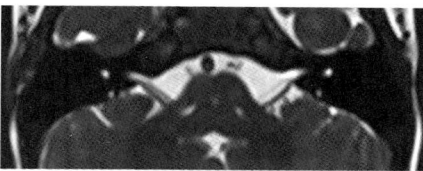

Fig. 10.2 Axial T2-weighted magnetic resonance imaging (MRI) showing narrow internal auditory canal.

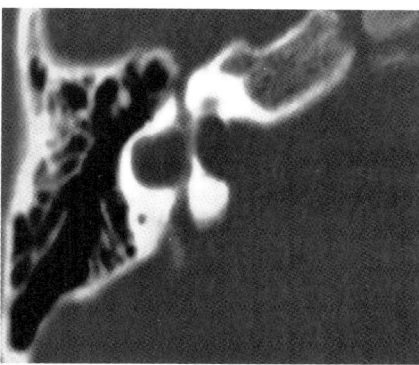

Fig. 10.3 Axial high-resolution computed tomography (HRCT) of temporal bone showing enlarged internal auditory canal.

- Owing to improvements in imaging technologies cochlear aperture should always be measured at mid-modiolar level.
- Stenosis of the IAC and cochlear aperture is associated with cochlear nerve deficiency, contraindicating cochlear implantation.
- Cochlear nerve can be aplastic, hypoplastic, or normal according to the diameter of the facial nerve.
  - Cochlear nerve is hypoplastic if cochlear nerve diameter is smaller than facial nerve diameter in sagittal cuts of magnetic resonance imaging (MRI).
  - If cochlear nerve is not seen in its compartment, then it is considered to be aplastic (**Fig. 10.4**).

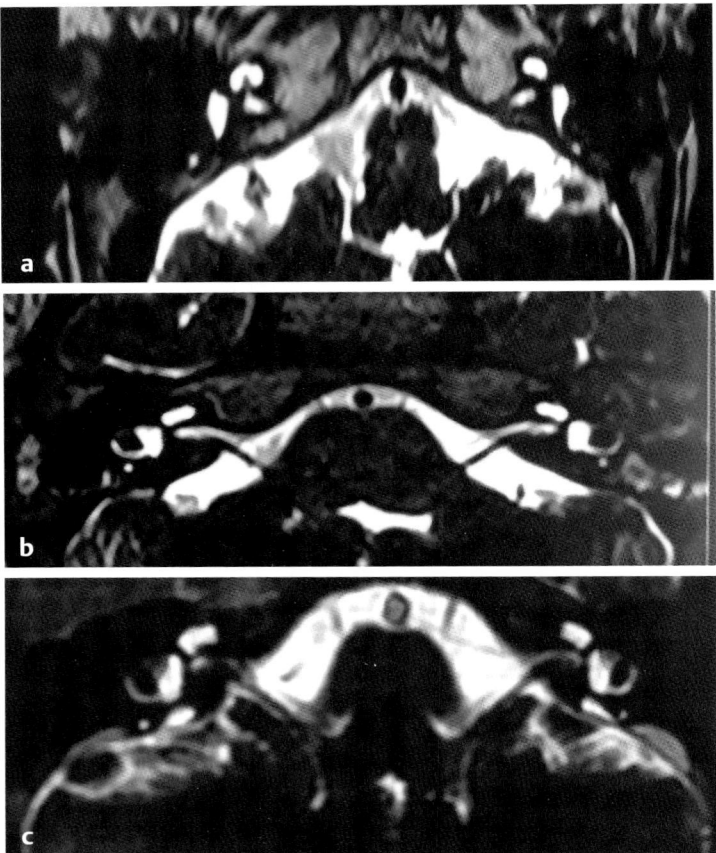

Fig. 10.4 (a–c) Axial T2-weighted magnetic resonance imaging (MRI) showing absent cochlear nerve.

- In cases of single-sided deafness, always look for deficiency of nerves.
    - There may be centers where only CT scan is done, and MRI is preferred if abnormalities of the IAC and fibrosis are seen.

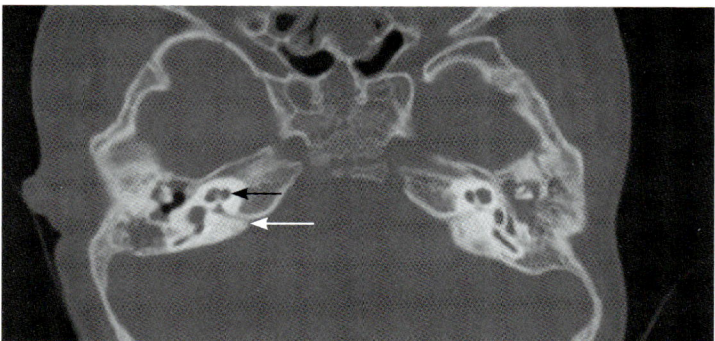

Fig. 10.5 Axial high-resolution computed tomography (HRCT) of temporal bone showing narrow internal auditory canal (*white arrow*) and narrow cochlear aperture (*black arrow*).

- I strongly suggest looking for cochlear aperture (it is bony cochlear nerve canal) along with the IAC measurements (**Fig. 10.5**).

Suggested Reading

Adunka OF, Roush PA, Teagle HF, et al. Internal auditory canal morphology in children with cochlear nerve deficiency. Otol Neurotol 2006;27(6):793–801

Buchman CA, Roush PA, Teagle HF, Brown CJ, Zdanski CJ, Grose JH. Auditory neuropathy characteristics in children with cochlear nerve deficiency. Ear Hear 2006;27(4):399–408

Jackler RK, Luxford WM, House WF. Congenital malformations of the inner ear: a classification based on embryogenesis. Laryngoscope 1987;97(3 Pt 2, Suppl 40):2–14

Sennaroglu L. Cochlear implantation in inner ear malformations—a review article. Cochlear Implants Int 2010;11(1):4–41

Sennaroğlu L, Özkan HB, Aslan F. Impact of cochleovestibular malformations in treating children with hearing loss. Cochlear I Science and Research Seminar; 2013; İstanbul, Turkey; pp. 23–27

Sennaroglu L, Ziyal I, Atas A, et al. Preliminary results of auditory brainstem implantation in prelingually deaf children with inner ear malformations including severe stenosis of the cochlear aperture and aplasia of the cochlear nerve. Otol Neurotol 2009;30(6):708–715

Valvassori GE, Palacios E. Magnetic resonance imaging of the internal auditory canal. Top Magn Reson Imaging 2000; 11(1):52–65

11 Impact of Intra-Operative X-Ray in Cochlear Implant

Introduction

The electrode array of cochlear implant is inserted into scala tympani in order to stimulate the spiral ganglion neurons.[1] The anatomy of cochlea and its tonotopic nature have ushered the evolution of various types of electrode arrays from single to multichannel, straight to curved, and lateral wall to medial wall.[2] Electrode array misplacement and misalignment are rare but serious complications in cochlear implant surgery. Any misalignment in positioning of electrode compromises the hearing spectrum of the patient. Extracochlear misplacement of electrode array has been reported in the internal acoustic meatus, eustachian tube, internal carotid artery, and superior semicircular canal. Even intracochlear misalignment of electrode array like under-insertion, tip fold over, kinking, and scalar migration are not uncommon and are often under-reported. Intraoperative radiograph taken during cochlear implant surgery is a quick, cheap, and noble technique to rule out these misalignments and misplacements. It also allows the opportunity to re-insert the mispositioned array before the weaning of anesthesia. Radiographs are an important document as the surgeon can fetch the postoperative X-ray anytime for medicolegal as well as for research purpose. These are important for:

- Incidence of electrode array misplacement and misalignment.
- Positioning methods for good view of electrode array inside cochlea.
- Assessment of electrode array positioning, depth, and integrity.

For cases of unilateral cochlear implant, cochlear view (modified Stenvers view) is done. In this view, to attain depth of electrode insertion X-ray beam is passed through the axis of modiolus, which is perpendicular to the basal turn of cochlea. Basal turn of cochlea is 45 degrees from mid-sagittal plane; therefore, patient's head is tilted 60 degrees away from operating ear and the operating table is tilted 15 degrees toward the operating ear. The X-ray beam is projected in an upward direction (from floor toward ceiling).

For bilateral implant, a transorbital (A-P) view is done where cochlea of both side can be visualized in one image. The patient is positioned in dorsal decubitus and the frame is placed under the head aligning the median sagittal plane in 90 degrees with the horizontal plane making sure that there is no head tilt or rotation.

The computer-assisted radio monitoring (C-arm) machine is covered with a sterile sheet to prevent inadvertent contamination. The image is immediately presented on the machine's screen and evaluated by the surgeon for the position and contour of the electrode. The approximate time taken for imaging and evaluation of the electrode position is 4 to 5 minutes. If the surgeon comes across any mispositioning, it is corrected immediately followed by a repeat X-ray. The radiograph is saved for future reference and documentation.

Incidence

Incidence varies from one study to another (1–8%).[3,4] The argument against routine radiograph to check electrode positioning includes radiation exposure, and purportedly there is low incidence of electrode misplacement. The practice of only performing radiograph when experiencing resistance during electrode insertion or in cases of anatomical abnormality can lead to low reporting of subtle misplacements and misalignments of electrode arrays such as tip fold overs, kinking, and loops. Neural response telemetry (NRT) alone cannot eliminate intracochlear misalignment of electrodes such as in tip fold over where the NRT can show on all electrodes. The extracochlear misplacements interpreted on radiographs can have normal responses on all electrodes in NRT.[5] The radiograph is superior to NRT in terms of confirming position of array, depth of insertion, proximity to modiolus, and presence of misalignment. With wrong positioning of head of the patient and X-ray beam, radiograph may be misinterpreted as electrode mispositioning and misalignment. Therefore, correct positioning of head of the patient is important because it strongly influences the orientation of the cochlea relative to X-ray projection and shows proper coiling of electrode array inside the cochlea (**Fig. 11.1a, b**).

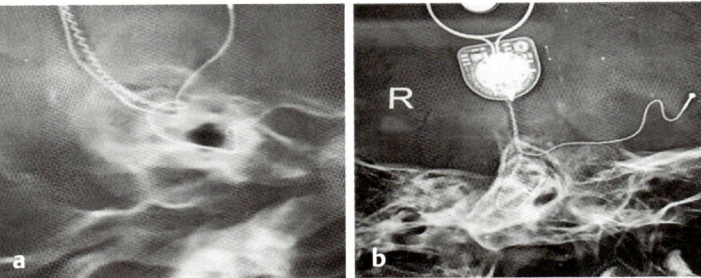

Fig. 11.1 **(a, b)** X-ray showing wrong positioning of head and X-ray beam.

Extracochlear Array Misplacement

Difficulties encountered during surgery such as poor visualization of anatomical landmarks, otosclerosis, cochlear anomalies especially incomplete partition (IP-III), and limited access increase the likelihood of misplacement. Inexperienced surgeons can mistake eustachian tube, subcochlear canaliculus and hypotympanic air cells as round window.

Kinking

Utmost gentleness and patience are required for electrode insertion. Resistance felt by the surgeon shortly after inserting the electrode array is due to array sliding against the cochlear wall but resistance after inserting two-thirds of array is an alarm for tip folding. Insertion of electrode even after resistance is the most common cause of kinking and tip fold over. Kinking is found to be most common with mentees. Tip fold over is less frequent and it can be missed if radiograph is not taken. Tip fold over can have normal responses on NRT (**Fig. 11.2a, b** and **Fig. 11.3**).

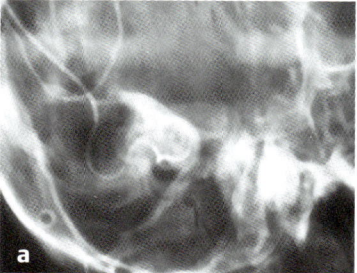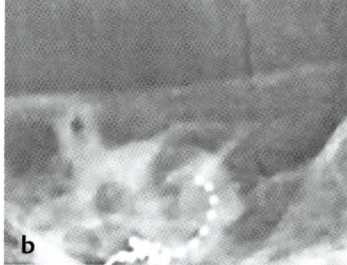

Fig. 11.2 **(a, b)** Modified Stenvers view showing kinking of electrode array.

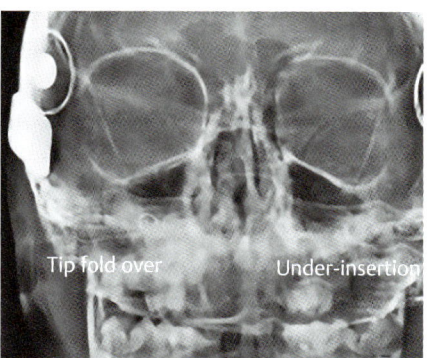

Fig. 11.3 Transorbital view of bilateral cochlear implant patient with tip folding in right cochlear electrode array and under-insertion on left side.

Under-insertion

The incidence of under-insertion is found more with the fellows and inexperienced surgeons. As electrodes are visible under microscope, the surgeon can visualize under-insertion by counting the number of electrodes outside the round window. Thus, under-insertion can be corrected easily on the operating table in the same sitting. NRT normally does not show response in electrodes lying outside the cochlea. Normal NRT was recorded in all electrodes with incomplete

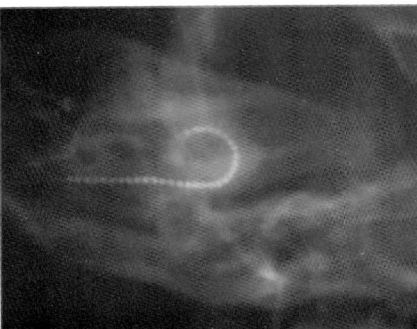

Fig. 11.4 Modified Stenvers view (cochlear view) of under-insertion of electrode.

insertion in 9.2% of cases.[6] This further reinforces the need to perform an intraoperative X-ray in cochlear implant surgeries (**Fig. 11.4**).

Electrophysiological Testing versus Radiograph

Electrophysiological testing like impedance and NRT provides information of individual electrode integrity as each electrode reads separately demonstrating its normal function.[2] Electrode can be misdirected into horizontal semicircular canal and can have near-normal impedance and NRT. This is hypothesized to be due to spread of current secondary to the high stimulation intensity which is similar to the response observed when the electrode array is placed in the cochlea.[5] Therefore, NRT solely does not eliminate intracochlear mispositioning of the electrode array but a radiograph can. Electric stimulation and responses are useful for determining the status of interface between the electrode and cochlea, but they cannot confirm the correct positioning of the electrode array.[2,5] Electrically evoked compound action potential (ECAP) can be recorded even for an extracochlear array. Air bubbles, blood clot, and bone dust around the electrode array can give false negative results.

Inherently, implantation on a bony structure carries the risk of mispositioning due to limited visibility; therefore, orthopedic surgeons routinely perform implantation under radiograph guidance. Cochlea is a bony structure with well-defined hollow membranous labyrinthine inside; it is connected to the middle cranial fossa via the internal auditory canal and semicircular canals through the vestibule. Due to proximity of structures and lack of visualization, electrodes can go into the nearby anatomical places like subcochlear canaliculus, eustachian tube, vestibule, internal auditory canal, semicircular canals, internal carotid artery, and middle ear cavity.[2] Perimodiolar electrode array can give deceptive appearance on imaging due to its curling nature.

Intraoperative radiograph during cochlear implant surgery is a quick, cheap, and noble technique to rule out misalignments and misplacements. Centers with routine cochlear implant surgery are recommended to have C-arm in operating room. We strongly recommend performing intraoperative radiograph in all cases irrespective of electrophysiological responses. It is a necessary tool for learning surgeons and is of utmost importance in cases of inner ear malformations.

References

1. Cartee LA, Miller CA, van den Honert C. Spiral ganglion cell site of excitation I: comparison of scala tympani and intrameatal electrode responses. Hear Res 2006;215(1-2):10–21
2. Ying Y-LM, Lin JW, Oghalai JS, Williamson RA. Cochlear implant electrode misplacement: incidence, evaluation, and management. Laryngoscope 2013;123(3):757–766

3. Dirr F, Hempel JM, Krause E, et al. Value of routine plain X-ray position checks after cochlear implantation. Otol Neurotol 2013;34(9):1666–1669

4. Cohen O, Sichel J-Y, Shaul C, Chen I, Roland JT, Perez R. The importance of intraoperative plain radiographs during cochlear implant surgery in patients with normal anatomy. Appl Sci (Basel) 2021;11(9):4144

5. Viccaro M, Covelli E, De Seta E, Balsamo G, Filipo R. The importance of intra-operative imaging during cochlear implant surgery. Cochlear Implants Int 2009;10(4):198–202

6. Coombs A, Clamp PJ, Armstrong S, Robinson PJ, Hajioff D. The role of post-operative imaging in cochlear implant surgery: a review of 220 adult cases. Cochlear Implants Int 2014;15(5):264–271

12 Interesting Imaging

This chapter brings forward some interesting radiological images of patients the author has encountered in the outpatient department (OPD) (**Fig. 12.1, Fig. 12.2, Fig. 12.3, Fig. 12.4, Fig. 12.5, Fig. 12.6, Fig. 12.7, Fig. 12.8,** and **Fig. 12.9**).

- Many times, the surgeon mistakes the subcochlear canaliculus for round window and the electrode array is inserted right into the petrous apex.

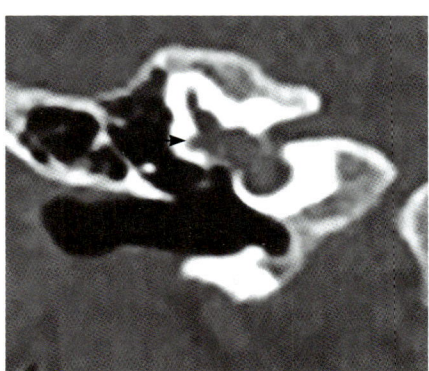

Fig. 12.1 Coronal high-resolution computed tomography (HRCT) scan of temporal bone showing dysplastic lateral semicircular canal (*black arrow*).

Note: If anomaly of lateral semicircular canal is found, be cautious about the facial nerve course.

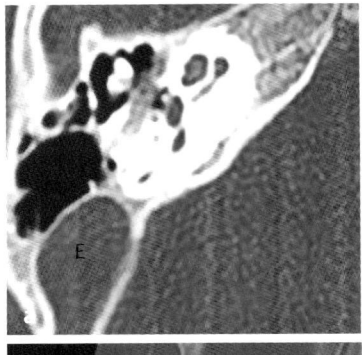
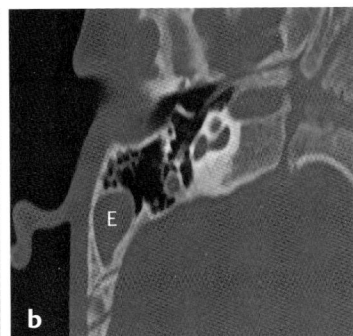
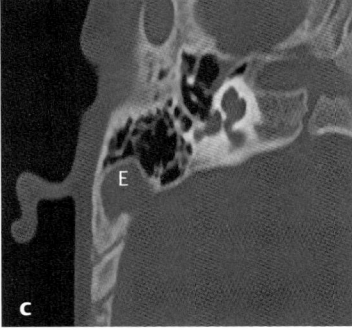

Fig. 12.2 (a–c) Axial high-resolution computed tomography (HRCT) scan of temporal bone showing emissary vein (E) filling up the antrum from sigmoid sinus.

Note: While drilling the mastoidectomy in cochlear implant, always see high-resolution computed tomography (HRCT) of temporal bone for low-lying dura, forward sigmoid sinus, and emissary vein.

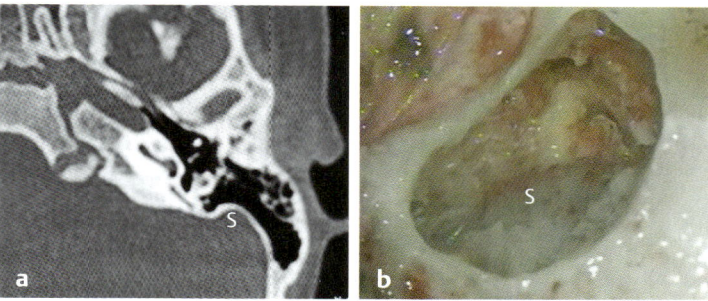

Fig. 12.3 **(a, b)** Image showing forward-lying sigmoid sinus.

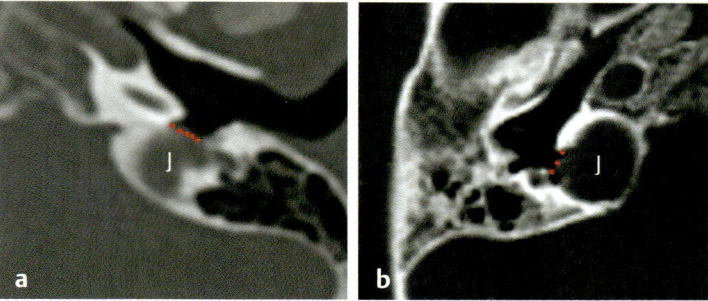

Fig. 12.4 **(a, b)** Axial computed tomography (CT) scan showing dehiscent jugular bulb (J) (*red dot*).

Note: During posterior tympanotomy one can injure jugular bulb lying in hypotympanum.

157

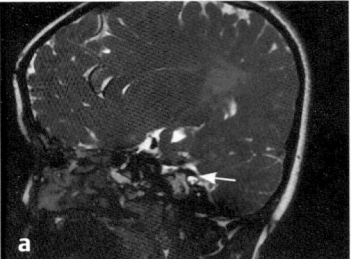
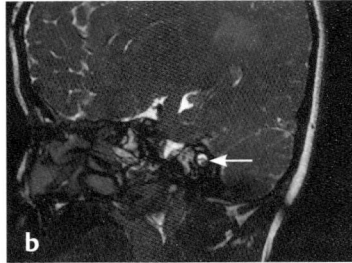

Fig. 12.5 **(a)** T2-weighted magnetic resonance imaging (MRI) showing the origin of facial nerve and vestibulocochlear nerve. **(b)** T2-weighted MRI showing all the four nerves. *White arrows* show the origin of nerves.

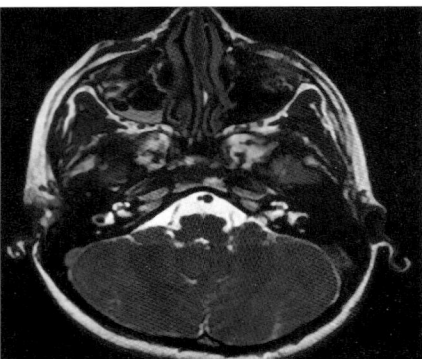

Fig. 12.6 Superior cerebellar artery vascular loop on right side with partial extension in internal auditory canal (IAC) for 2 to 3 mm abutting nerves.

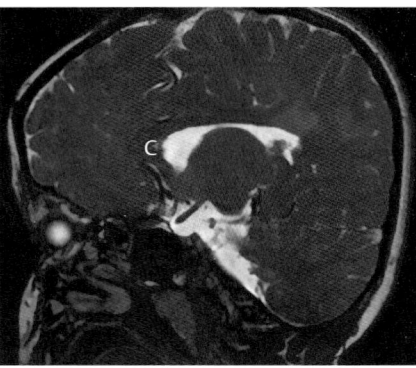

Fig. 12.7 T2-weighted magnetic resonance imaging (MRI) showing abnormal signal in splenium of corpus callosum, adjacent white matter, and right central semi-ovale suggestive of congenital infection.

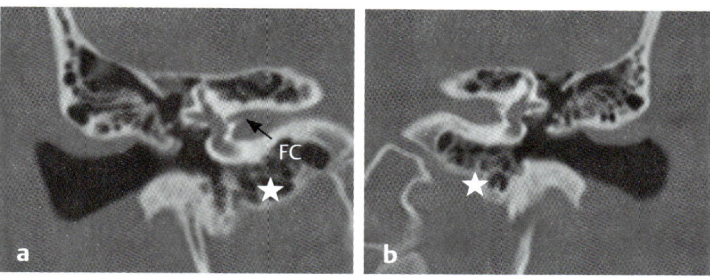

Fig. 12.8 Coronal computed tomography (CT) scan showing subcochlear canaliculus (*white star*) and falciform crest.

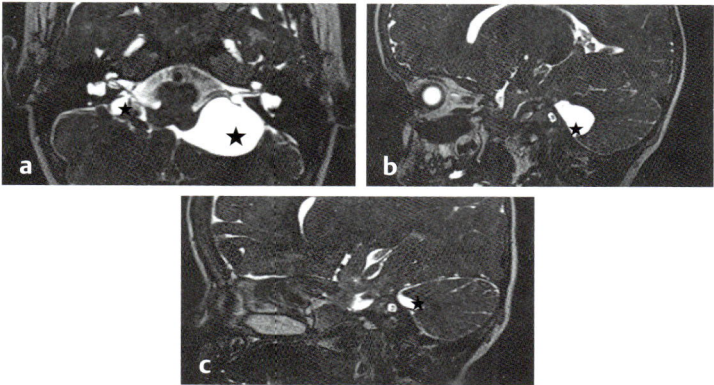

Fig. 12.9 T2-weighted magnetic resonance imaging (MRI). **(a)** Axial section showing arytenoid cyst (*black star*) abutting the internal auditory canal (IAC). **(b, c)** Sagittal section of the same patient, left and right respectively.

Note: Case of arytenoid cyst abutting the internal auditory canal is an incidental finding. Cochlear implant can be done in these patients without any complications.

Case
Subtotal Petrosectomy

Operated case of cholesteatoma with canal wall up done 4 years back. The patient presented in outpatient department 2 years back with profound sensory neural hearing loss and with mild recurrence of disease (**Fig. 12.10, Fig. 12.11, Fig. 12.12, Fig. 12.13, Fig. 12.14,** and **Fig. 12.15**).

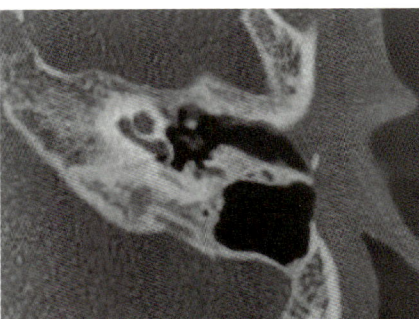

Fig. 12.10 Axial high-resolution computed tomography (HRCT) scan of temporal bone post mastoidectomy.

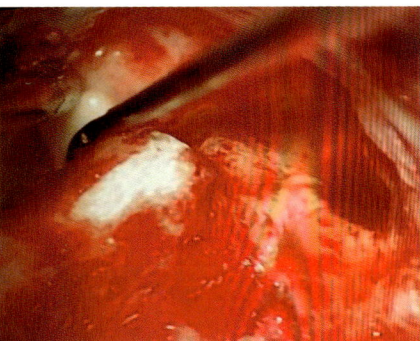

Fig. 12.11 Intraoperative picture of disease clearance.

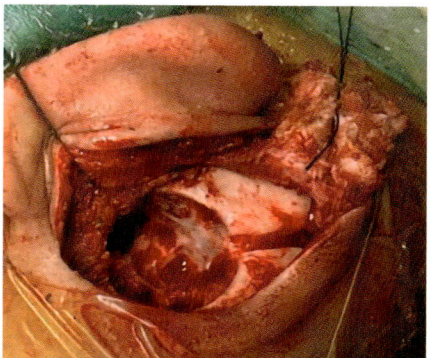

Fig. 12.12 Intraoperative picture showing clearance of cells with canal wall down done.

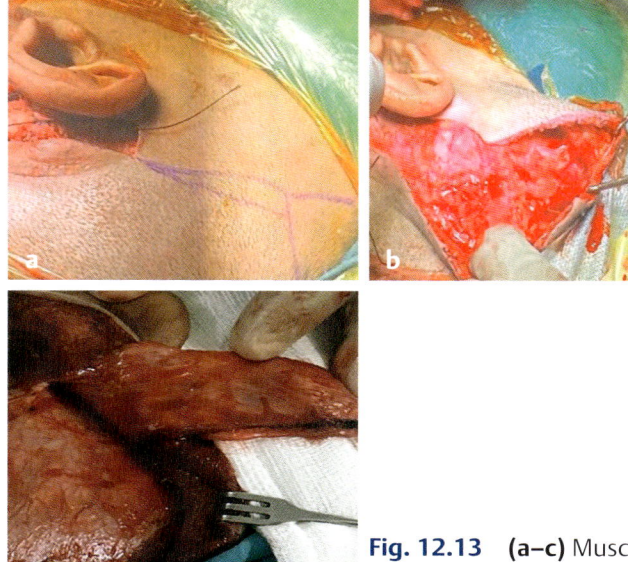

Fig. 12.13 **(a–c)** Muscle flap creation.

161

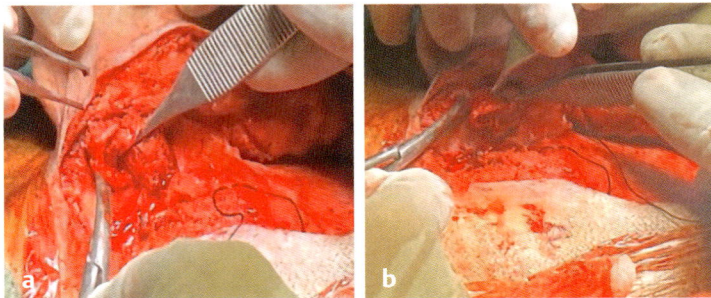

Fig. 12.14 **(a, b)** Occlusion of external auditory canal.

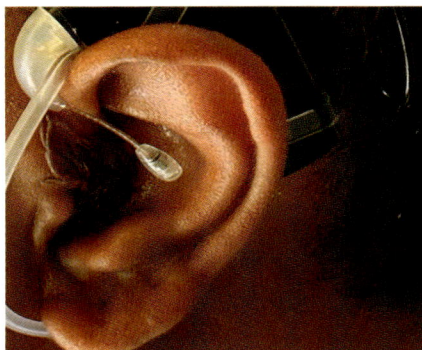

Fig. 12.15 Postoperative picture of subtotal petrosectomy after 1 year of surgery.

Magnet Displacement

Magnet displacement occurs occasionally due to fall down (there is always a history associated with trauma). These children normally come with a history of processor falling down from its position. An X-ray helps in identifying the cause (**Fig.12.16**).

Note: When patients complain of device not being retained at the receiver stimulator site along with a history of fall, look for magnet displacement.

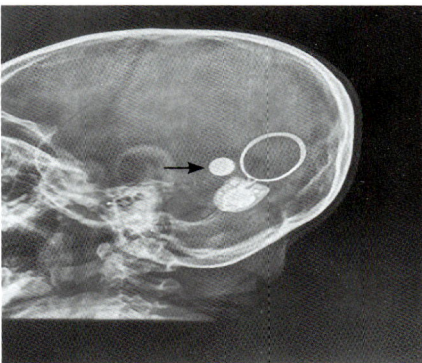

Fig. 12.16 X-ray Stenvers view showing displacement of magnet (*black arrow*).

13 Difficult Cochlear Implant Cases

Cochlear Implantation in Blood Disorders

An 11-month-old child after all routine preoperative evaluation was posted for right side cochlear implantation. The preoperative evaluation at our hospital includes audiological tests, computed tomography (CT) and magnetic resonance imaging (MRI) of cochlea, and blood parameters— complete hemogram, liver and renal function tests, bleeding time, clotting time, and prothrombin time. After obtaining preoperative fitness from pediatric and anesthesia department, the patient underwent right side implant surgery under general anesthesia. The intraoperative and immediate postoperative periods were uneventful. After 36 hours of surgery the child started developing right periorbital ecchymosis (**Fig. 13.1**). We suspected tight bandage as the cause for black eye and the same was loosened. But the child developed ecchymosis around left eye after 42 hours of surgery with the development of hematoma over the right scalp region (**Fig. 13.2**).

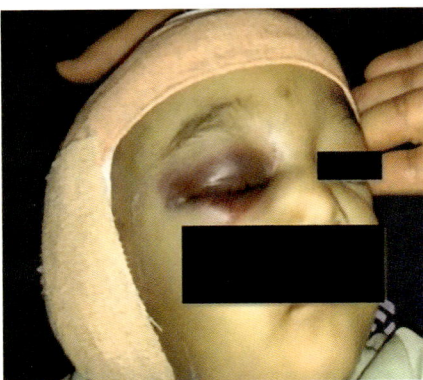

Fig. 13.1 Right periorbital ecchymosis after 36 hours of ipsilateral cochlear implant.

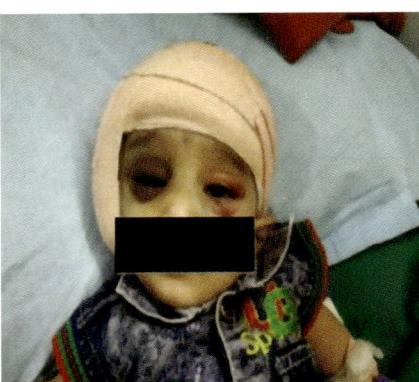

Fig. 13.2 The child developed bilateral periorbital ecchymosis after 42 hours of surgery.

The child was taken into operating room and the surgical wound exploration was done, but no bleeding points were found. The wound was closed, and mastoid dressing applied. Within half hour, soakage of dressing was noted. At this stage we suspected an undiagnosed coagulation disorder, and all the blood parameters were repeated. The hemoglobin level fell to 4.2 g/dL from the preoperative value of 10.8 g/dL.

The bleeding time, clotting time, and prothrombin time were normal. The activated partial thromboplastin time (aPTT) was also advised, and it was found to be deranged (control was 25–30 seconds). A hematology opinion was taken in view of deranged aPTT, and it was advised to rule out clotting factor deficiency. The patient was transfused with one unit of packed red blood cells (PRBC) and two units of fresh frozen plasma (FFP) and in the meantime the wound was re-explored to make sure that no active bleeders were missing. On re-exploration, blood clots with diffuse ooze from the periosteal plane were noted. Surgicel was kept over periosteum and wound closed in layers. Factor IX was found to be deficient, and a diagnosis of hemophilia B was made. Factor IX concentrates were procured, and the dose administered intravenously was 1200 units as bolus and 600 units every day thereafter. The child's hematoma and periorbital ecchymosis started resolving with increase in hemoglobin levels and normalization of aPPT value. The child was discharged on postoperative day 10 after suture removal. The child is on regular follow-up (**Fig. 13.3**).

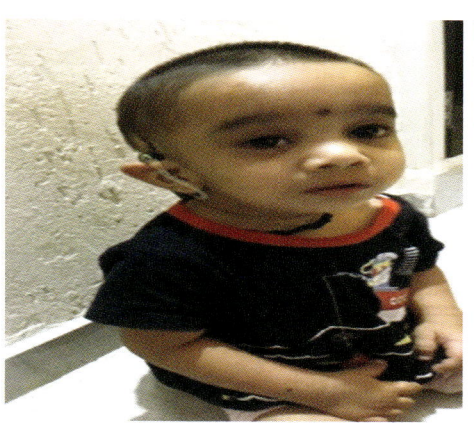

Fig. 13.3 The child with behind-the-ear processor undergoing rehabilitation.

Our Hospital Protocol for Perioperative and Postoperative Management of Hemophilia B Patients

aPTT is now mandatory for all cochlear implant patients. In diagnosed cases of hemophilia B a loading dose of Factor IX with dosage of 100 to 120 units/kg in normal saline is administered intravenously. The subsequent doses (approximately half of the loading dose) are to be given at an interval equal to the half-life of the product used. The patient should be under close monitoring with serial measurements of coagulation parameters and dose adjustment accordingly.

Case 2
Cochlear Implant Revision Cases

Cochlear implantation, which is considered to be a safe surgical procedure, is uncommonly found to be associated with infection at the implant site many months or years after the surgery. One of the reasons for this is the formation of biofilms at the implant site.

Biofilms is a structured aggregate of bacteria that are attached to an inert or living surface in an irreversible manner embedded in a matrix of extracellular polymeric substances. These bacterial colonies exist in a subclinical state, producing endotoxins and exotoxins. The biofilm-producing organisms along with their toxins create a proinflammatory state leading to chronic inflammation. It is uncommon for cochlear implants to be complicated by microbial infection. Rarely, cochlear implant can be a site for harboring biofilm-producing organisms. The complications arising out of this can be hematoma, discharging sinus or fistulas, and necrosis (**Fig. 13.4**). It is difficult to treat these conditions as biofilm

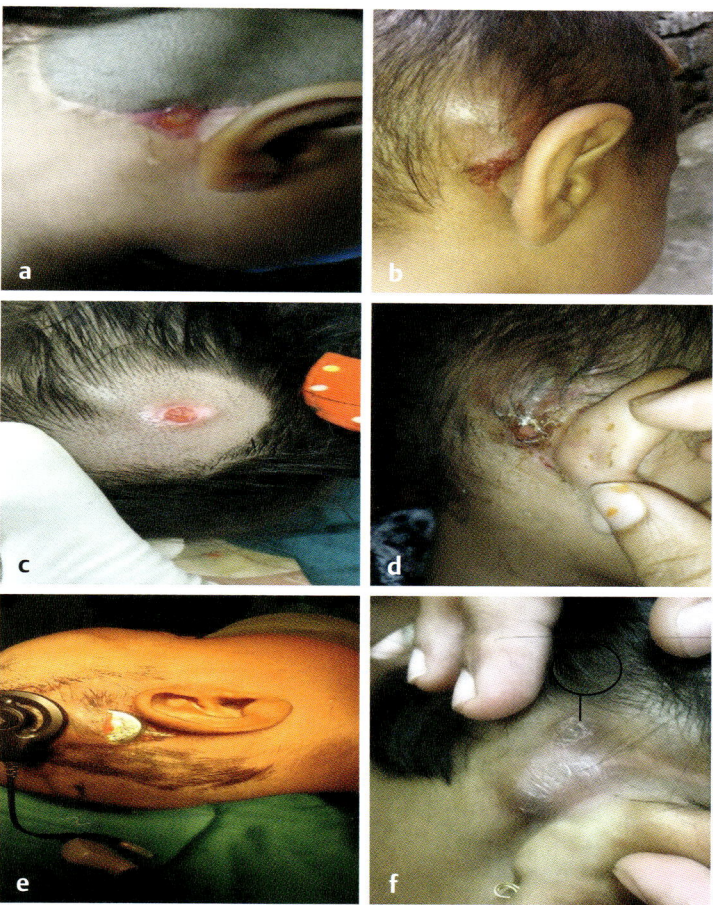

Fig. 13.4 **(a–f)** Various biofilm-related complications at cochlear implant site.

is notorious for having antimicrobial resistance to common antibiotics and may require explanting the cochlear implant.

Till date there has been no straightforward guidelines to deal with biofilm infection. However, interventional

169

strategies include removal of infected bodies and meticulous debridement.

How We Do It?

- Perform wide local excision of the affected site (**Fig. 13.5**).
- Expose the cochlear implant.
- Remove the magnet from the pocket and immerse the implant body in 6% hydrogen peroxide for 1 hour (**Fig. 13.6**).
- Then treat the magnet with 6% hydrogen peroxide and polyhexanide solution.
- After half an hour dip, put the implant body in polyhexanide and betaine surfactant for half hour.
- Fill the mastoid cavity with polyhexanide and betaine solution, ensuring electrode array is not out of cochlea while manipulating the implant body.
- Debride the suspected biofilm.
- Drill a new bed and tunnel.

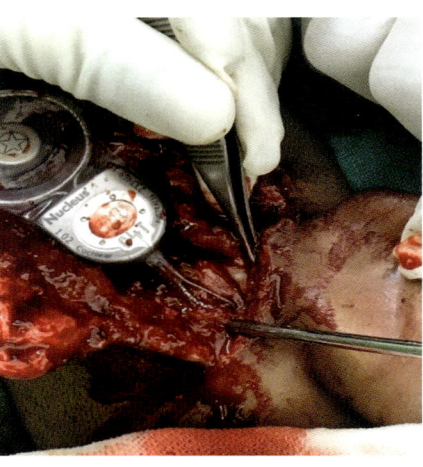

Fig. 13.5 Wide excision of the swelling shown in **Fig. 13.4**.

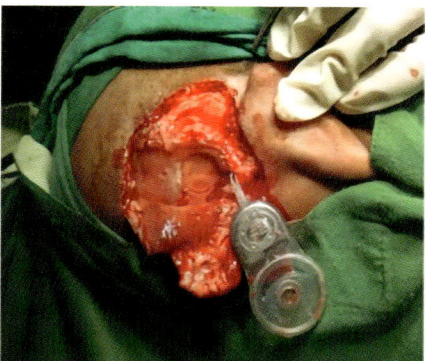

Fig. 13.6 The implant after magnet was removed and treated with anti-biofilm agents.

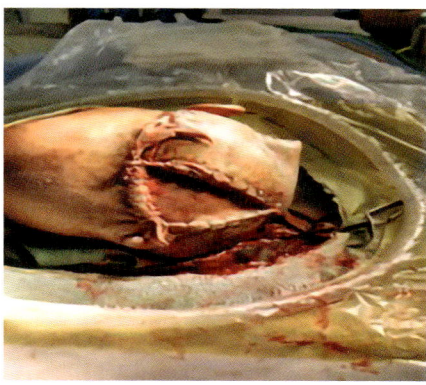

Fig. 13.7 Closure of the surgical site using local tissue flap.

- Prepare double-layered vascularized soft tissue local flap (**Fig. 13.7**).
- After repositing the implant body and magnet, change the cochleostomy site packing periosteal tissue.
- Before closure, the mastoid cavity is filled with an anti-biofilm agent and polyhexanide gel is applied on the bed as well as flap cover.
- Neural response telemetry (NRT) is done to check the normal functioning of the implant.

171

- Postoperatively, inject Augmentin (50–60 mg/kg/day) and inject piperacillin–tazobactam (200–300 mg/kg/day) for 10 days followed by oral antibiotics for a week and oral rifampicin (10 mg/kg/day) for 6 months (**Fig. 13.8** and **Fig. 13.9**).
- Histopathological examination of the excised tissues is performed.

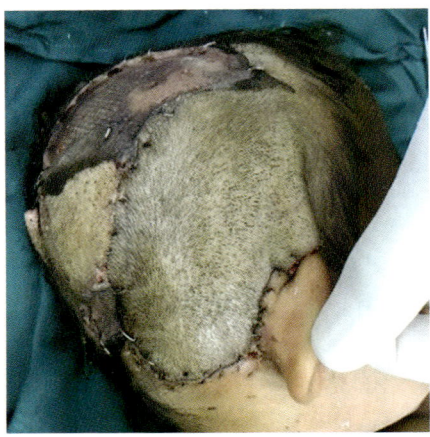

Fig. 13.8 Postoperative day 10 of the local flap in **Fig. 13.7**.

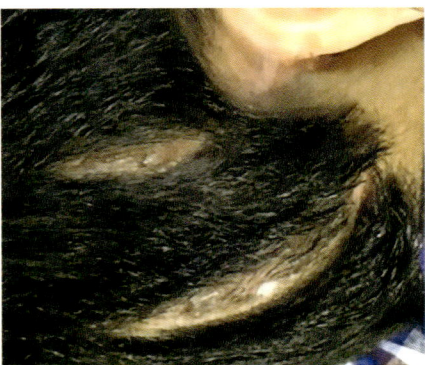

Fig. 13.9 After 1 year with no signs of infection.

Case 3
Magnet Displacement

A patient presented with a history of falling of behind-the-ear processor from the head very often. On detailed history taking, we found the patient had a history of head trauma. X-ray in modified Stenvers view was done to confirm the position of the implant. The magnet was found to be displaced from its site and surgery was planned (**Fig. 13.10**). The preoperative options were either the same magnet is to be replaced or place a new magnet.

After surgical site painting and draping, incision was made at the site, skin and subcutaneous tissues were incised, and after careful dissection (taking care not to injure the receiver stimulator titanium case) the magnet was placed in its position. Utmost care was taken during surgery as the magnet gets attracted to all the instruments and can fall down from the surgical field. The wound was closed in two layers (**Fig. 13.11, Fig. 13.12,** and **Fig. 13.13**).

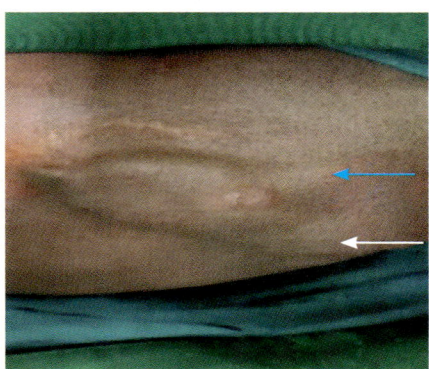

Fig. 13.10   The displaced magnet site (*white arrow*) and the original site (*blue arrow*).

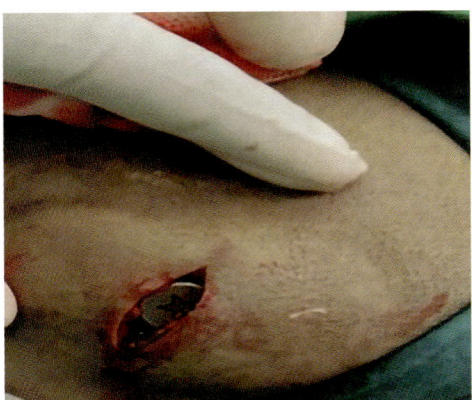

Fig. 13.11 Surgical incision.

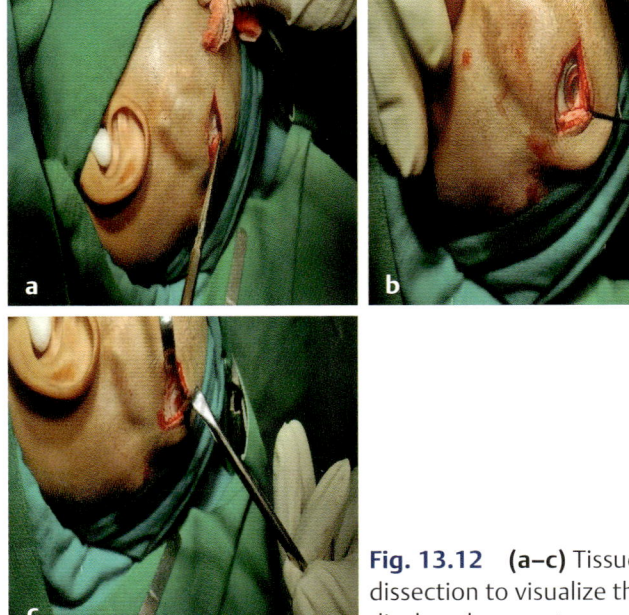

Fig. 13.12 **(a–c)** Tissue dissection to visualize the displaced magnet.

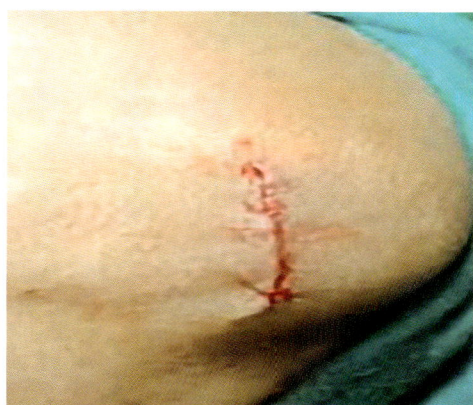

Fig. 13.13 Surgical incision closure.

Case 4
Facial Nerve at Abnormal Location

Preoperative high-resolution computed tomography (HRCT) of a patient planned for cochlear implantation showed ossicles at an abnormal location with anomalous course of the facial nerve (**Fig. 13.14**).

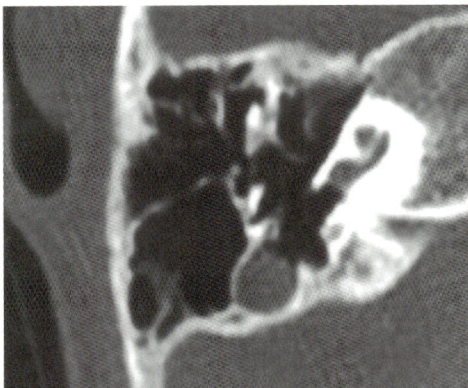

Fig. 13.14 High-resolution computed tomography (HRCT) of temporal bone axial section showing incus and facial nerve at the aditus region.

Intraoperative Finding

When the aditus was opened, the facial nerve was found lying in the aditus region with the incus and stapes at abnormal location. Posterior tympanotomy was done. The round window was visualized with 1 to 2 mm drilling of posterior tympanotomy (**Fig. 13.15**).

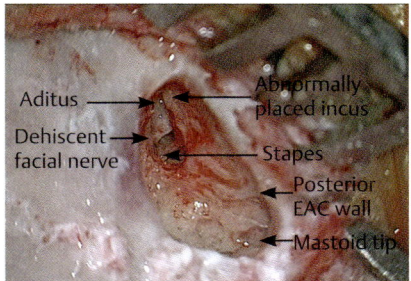

Fig. 13.15 Intraoperative findings. External auditory canal (EAC).

Index